I0786824

EXERCISE

SMART

U.K. Edition

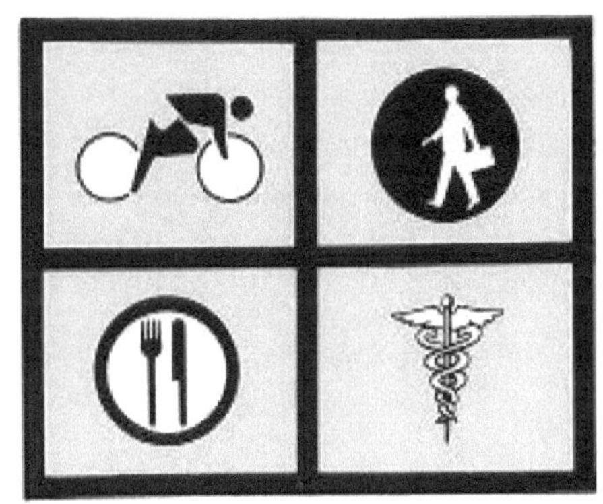

Earl Simmons

NoPaperPress™

CONTENTS

5. LIFE-LONG FITNESS

TABLES

FIGURES

1. BEING FIT IS CRUCIAL

The person we call moderately active today, that is someone who walks an hour everyday and engages in some sport on the weekend, would have been considered sedentary a century ago! In many countries, the general lack of fitness of countless adults, who begin to show signs of old age – shortness of breath, obesity and clogged arteries – years earlier than their counterparts of just a few generations ago, is considered a national problem. The unfit person, who wants to call it a day two hours before quitting time and is obsessed with minor aches and pains, often lacks the vigor and physical toughness to cope with the long hours and high-stress that are part of the 21st century. The fit person, on the other hand, typically has greater energy, tackles problems and projects head on, gets more done in less time, is better able to cope with stress, has a positive approach that is contagious, and does not get sick as often.

In our view, for a person to fully enjoy life he or she must manage their health as effectively as they manage the other aspects of their life – and that this is best done using tried and true management techniques: first, define the problem; second, obtain the relevant facts; third, formulate an action plan; and last, make it happen! That is precisely the approach taken in this book. The intent here is to provide in a relatively complete form the facts needed for an in-depth understanding of all the components of an exercise program, and then to demonstrate how the information can be used to plan and implement a successful personal exercise routine. To do this in the most efficient manner, the following pages are organized along the lines of an exercise handbook – with the emphasis on facts not frills – and all with the busy adult in mind.

Medical personnel, health education specialists, personal fitness trainers, and corporate fitness directors should find the data in this eBook useful in devising or supervising physical fitness programs. Whether this book is used as a professional reference, or as a personal exercise guide, the aim is to provide the facts and data needed to achieve and maintain a healthful physical fitness level.

Four of the leading causes of death in the United States are heart disease, cancer, stroke and diabetes. That's the bad news. The good news is that

research indicates that people who exercise regularly, who eat the right foods and who maintain a normal weight, i.e., who are physically fit, can reduce their risk of heart attack, stroke and diabetes, and also gain some protection against certain forms of cancer.

Cardiovascular System

More than 700 million people world wide have some form of cardiovascular disease. According to the American Heart Association, cardiovascular disease claims the lives of more than two million people every year, surprisingly almost half are women, and many of the victims are relatively young. Because of this, some knowledge of the workings and diseases of the cardiovascular system is appropriate before we begin to discuss physical fitness.

As illustrated in Figure 1.1, the cardiovascular system consists of the blood vessels through which blood flows and the heart which produces this flow. Beating about 72 times per minute, the average heart pumps approximately two ounces of blood per beat, resulting in a blood flow rate of somewhat more than one gallon per minute. The left side of the heart discharges oxygen-rich blood through the arteries bringing nourishment and oxygen to the body's cells. After waste gases such as carbon dioxide are removed from the cells, veins return the blood to the right side of the heart. The heart then pumps the blood to the lungs where carbon dioxide is removed and oxygen is absorbed from the air we breathe. The cycle is completed as the left side of the heart receives this oxygen-rich blood. When something goes wrong with the system, the condition is called cardiovascular disease.

Cardiovascular disease comes in many forms: the heart muscle can fail or become infected; valves can leak or refuse to close when they should; the timing mechanism can become erratic; but the most pervasive killers are high blood pressure and atherosclerosis.

Hypertension

Recognized as a health problem of the first magnitude, hypertension – also called high blood pressure – is perhaps the most common cardiovascular disease, afflicting more than 45 million adults in the United States. The dangers of hypertension include heart failure, heart attack, a rupture of major blood vessels in the brain (stroke), clotting in major arteries, eye problems and impairment of kidney function.

Simply stated, blood pressure is the force per unit area exerted by blood

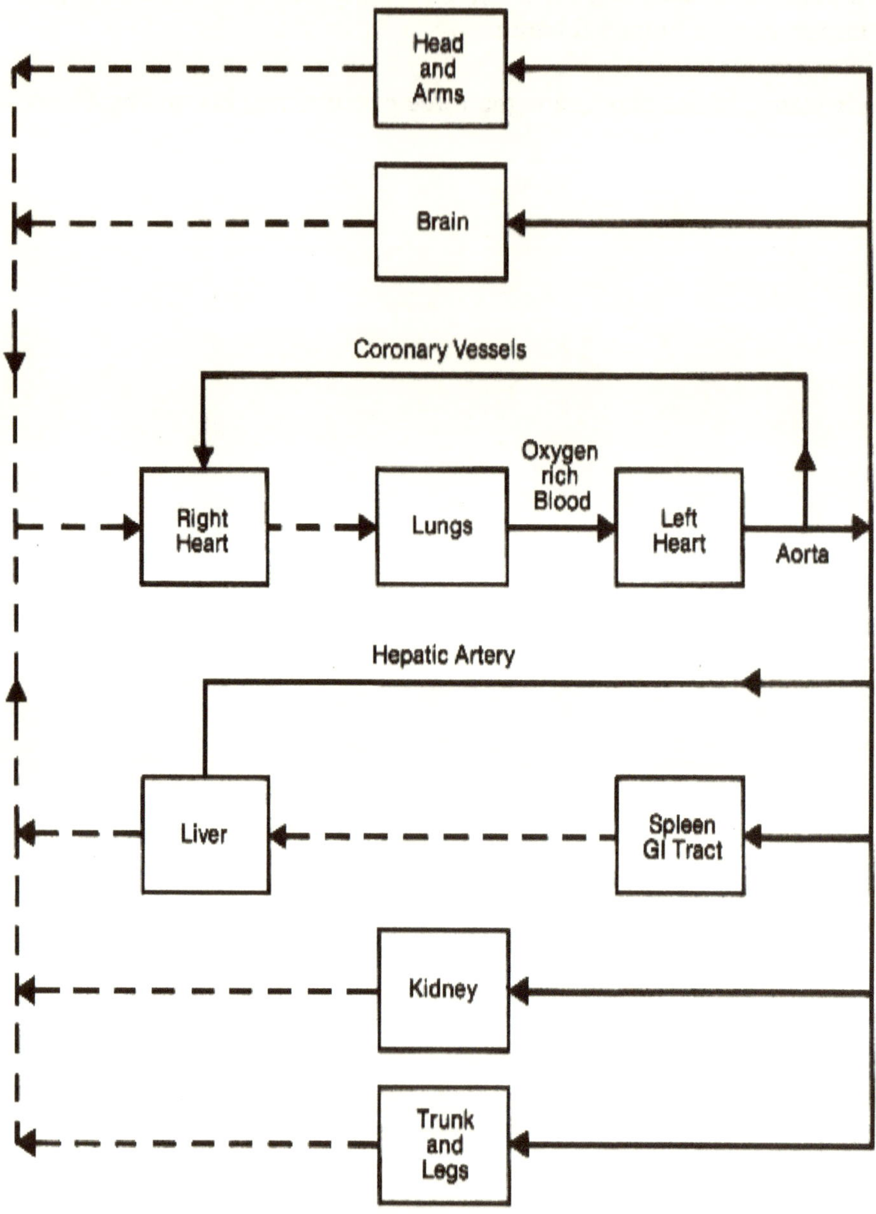

Figure 1.1: Block Diagram of Cardiovascular System

10

against the walls of the blood vessels and heart. Blood pressure is usually recorded as two readings: an upper, or systolic figure, and a lower, or diastolic figure. As the heart contracts, blood pressure rises to the systolic level, and each time the heart relaxes the pressure falls to the diastolic level. A person has high blood pressure, or hypertension, when their blood pressure reaches 130 systolic or 80 diastolic (130/80) and persistently remains at that level or higher. At this point medical attention is indicated.

Recent studies, however, have shown that artery damage and increased risk of cardiovascular disease can begin at blood pressure levels that were previously thought to be normal. The National Heart, Lung and Blood Institute now uses the term "prehypertension," defined as blood pressure that is higher than 130 millimeters of mercury systolic or higher than 80 millimeters of mercury diastolic. This new category includes an unknown number of more people. The National Heart, Lung and Blood Institute's position is that people with blood pressure readings in this range do not have high blood pressure yet and do not need to take medication - but are likely to develop high blood pressure and should try to lower their pressure through lifestyle changes, such as a change in diet, exercise or losing weight.

Approximately 85 percent of those diagnosed with high blood pressure have what is called "primary hypertension," also called "essential hypertension." This designation refers to the group of hypertension cases for which there is no apparent explanation. If left untreated, primary hypertension greatly increases the risk that other cardiovascular diseases will occur. Although there is no cure for primary hypertension, it can be controlled – most often with medication.

The remaining 15 percent of those with high blood pressure have what is called "secondary hypertension." This form of high blood pressure can be attributed to a specific cause, such as clogged arteries or kidney disease. If the underlying cause of secondary hypertension can be diagnosed and eliminated, often secondary hypertension can be cured.

In most cases, high blood pressure is painless and produces no symptoms. If symptoms do occur, they are similar to those caused by a myriad of other disorders. Because of this, even though high blood pressure is quite prevalent, it is discovered most often during the course of a periodic medical examination. Some cases of hypertension can be managed effectively through a change in diet alone – without drugs. For the overweight,

physicians first usually recommend a reducing diet. This is because the heart of an obese person is strained, being forced to pump more blood volume through a much larger cardiovascular system. Most doctors also urge that salt, more properly
sodium, be restricted to curb the body's retention of fluid, thereby decreasing the volume of blood that must be pumped. If lifestyle changes fail to reduce a person's blood pressure, medication is usually prescribed.

Atherosclerosis

The narrowing and blocking of the blood vessels by the build-up of fatty deposits and other materials is called atherosclerosis, also known as hardening of the arteries.

The heart is a muscle and needs blood to survive. Narrowing of the blood vessels to the point where there is a decrease in the blood supply to the heart can cause angina (chest pain). The total absence of flow in a coronary artery leading to the heart, called a coronary occlusion or a coronary thrombosis, can damage or cause the death of a piece of the heart muscle, which cardiologists call a myocardial infarction or heart attack.

Heart Attack Warning Signs

- Prolonged, oppressive pain or unusual discomfort in the center of the chest.

- Pain may spread to shoulder, arm, neck or jaw, and sweating, nausea, vomiting and shortness of breath may ensue.

Sometimes the symptoms subside, then return. If these warning signs are experienced, it is important to act quickly. If a doctor is not immediately available, get to a hospital emergency room at once.

Risk Factors Leading to Cardiovascular Disease

The rate of cardiovascular disease in the United States is much higher than that of most industrialized nations. In fact, the death rate for men in the U.S. ages 45 to 54 years is the second highest among the world's richest countries. Started in 1948, the "Framingham Study," under the direction of the National Heart Institute, examined thousands of people and demonstrated a clear statistical association between cardiovascular disease and a number of "risk factors." These risk factors have been found time and time again in the medical history of thousands of people who have had heart attacks.

First, there are the risk factors we cannot control: gender and heredity. The data clearly show that men have heart attacks earlier and more frequently than women; that pre-menopausal women are almost immune to heart attacks; that individuals with a family history of premature heart disease have a far greater risk than those whose ancestors lived to a ripe old age; and that diabetes (left untreated) increases the danger of heart disease.

The **risk factors** often attributed to our lifestyle and, therefore, under our control – at least to some extent – are in approximate order of importance:

- **High blood pressure left untreated.**

- **Cigarette smoking.**

- **High blood cholesterol and other blood fats.**

- **Obesity.**

- **Lack of physical activity.**

- **A high-pressure existence.**

No one of these factors has been called the single cause of cardiovascular disease. Indeed studies show that a combination of risk factors dramatically increases the danger.

Stroke

Although some cells in the body can survive for as long as fifty minutes without blood, if the flow to the brain is cut off for ten or twenty seconds unconsciousness will occur, and deprived of blood circulation for four minutes or more results in brain damage. Blockage of the blood vessels leading to the brain or in the brain itself (sometimes a manifestation of atherosclerosis, other times caused by a clot) is called stroke.

Stroke Warning Signs

- Sudden numbness or weakness of the face, arm or leg, especially on one side

- Sudden headache, confusion, trouble speaking or understanding

- Sudden trouble seeing in one or both eyes

- Sudden trouble walking, dizziness, loss of balance or coordination

Stroke and cardiovascular disease have a lot in common: High blood pressure is an important cause of both illnesses, and many of the preceding cardiovascular disease risk factors also apply to stroke.

Diabetes

With the ranks of the obese increasing dramatically, the incidence of diabetes is reaching epidemic proportions in the United States - posing a somber threat to our nation's well being. In 2002, diabetes was the fifth leading cause of non-accidental death in the United States. Type 2 diabetes is the most common form. Previously called adult-onset diabetes, type-2 diabetes can begin at any age. It usually starts with insulin resistance, a condition in which fat, muscle, and liver cells do not use insulin properly. Being overweight and inactive (read unfit) increases your chance of developing type 2 diabetes.

What Can be Done?

It is not possible stop cardiovascular disease, heart attacks, stroke and diabetes completely, but enough is known to prevent many - if not most - premature incidents. In the pages that follow, a program will be outlined with specific lifestyle modifications and exercise recommendations that are remarkably simple.

(Note, the cancer battle is not as straight forward. Substantial evidence indicates the fitness prescription that reduces the risk of cardiovascular disease, stroke and diabetes also exhibits a benefit against certain malignances, such as colon cancer and breast cancer, and a promising benefit against others, but offers no protection with regard to many other cancers.)

➡ Note that the material in this book is not intended as a substitute for medical counseling. Everyone should have a medical checkup before beginning a physical fitness program (whether the program involves exercise, nutritional changes, or weight loss). Moreover, the physician conducting the medical exam should be made fully aware of and should approve the specific physical fitness routine planned. Further, the reader is cautioned that all fitness programs include some risk of injury or illness.

2. HOW TO BECOME FIT

The physical conditions and living habits that increase the risk of premature heart disease, stroke and diabetes have been identified, but for every risk there is a counteracting step you can take. Said another way, to reduce your risk you need to look at your entire way of living and in some instances rearrange your priorities.

No one set of rules will guarantee health or fitness. Age, gender, and physical condition are all factors in determining the specific program that is best for you. We can delineate, however, the general guidelines for a total program:

- ☐ **Have periodic medical checkups.**

- ☐ **Do not smoke.**

- ☐ **Exercise regularly.**

- ☐ **Practice good nutritional habits.**

- ☐ **Maintain a proper weight level.**

- ☐ **Learn to relax.**

- ☐ **Drink alcoholic beverages in moderation – if at all.**

Do Not Smoke!

Warning: The Surgeon General has determined that cigarette smoking is dangerous to your health! These facts are not disputed: nicotine and carbon monoxide in tobacco smoke are pathologically related to cardiovascular disease; and tar collects in the pulmonary passages leading the way to emphysema and lung cancer. Clearly, tobacco and physical fitness are mutually exclusive. Undoubtedly, one of the best things you can do for your body is to stop smoking.

Learn to Relax

Some researchers contend that the greatest single contributor to the development of coronary risk factors is the presence of a "TYPE-A, coronary personality." Such individuals are aggressive, competitive, compulsive, impatient, work additive and frequently anxious. These obsessions can lead to excessive social drinking – and often to domestic turmoil.

It is not easy to avoid stressful situations in the pressure-cooker world that is the 21st century. Although some stress is a normal, even a healthy part of living, sometimes you may be so stressed by work or worry that you simply cannot relax. When this happens, you need a calming regulator for your emotions. Some people have a built in defense that says "Calm Down!" Others may benefit from a change of pace, such as a workout at the fitness facility, a brisk walk, or a relaxing talk with a friend or advisor.

The Benefits of Being Fit

Although our primary aim is to reduce the risk of cardiovascular illness, stroke, cancer and diabetes, physical fitness is much more than not being sick or merely being well. It is a positive quality. Ideally, it is the ability to withstand stress, and to persevere under circumstances where an unfit person would quit.

While the results will differ from individual to individual, most often **being fit will result in a longer life expectancy, less illness, a healthful appearance, the ability to work (and play) with vigor and an energy reserve for emergencies.**

After a prolonged period of sedentary living, people, who undertake a physical fitness program and attain a heightened level of fitness, report a dramatic reduction in chronic fatigue, an improved ability to relax, more energy for day-to-day tasks, firmer muscles and increased strength. In short, they feel better and look better too!

Everyone knows regular exercise improves your strength and flexibility and can help you lose weight. But did you know that regular exercise promotes the lose of fat rather than muscle and other nonfat tissue? Research also shows that people who include regular exercise as part of their weight-lose program are more likely to keep off the weight they have lost than people who only changed their diet.

Not so evident, but perhaps even more important, are the beneficial changes in the functioning of the heart, lungs and circulatory system. Physical activity lowers your risk of developing heart disease and helps control blood pressure and diabetes. In addition, the old-fashioned idea that exercise is bad for the heart has been shown to be without scientific foundation. The heart is a pump made of muscle. Just as exercise strengthens the other muscles in your body, it also strengthens your heart. With exercise your heart beat becomes stronger and steadier, breathing becomes deeper, and circulation improves.

In more specific terms, a well-designed total fitness program – encompassing exercise, nutrition and weight control – will:

- Help you lose weight

- Lower your blood pressure

- Make your heart stronger and more efficient

- Keep your arteries supple and young

- Speed up your basal metabolism

- Convert fat to muscle

- Make your muscles larger with more definition - and more powerful

- Strengthen your bones

In addition, being fit will also reduce your risk of:

- Cardiovascular disease

- Stroke

- High blood pressure

- Diabetes

- Certain cancers

- Osteoporosis and bone fractures

Longevity: Being fit can't quite turn back the clock but it can make you look and feel younger than your chronological age – and you will probably live longer too. There are a number of scientific studies that have concluded that regular exercise reduces the hardship of illness and disability in old age and actually prolongs life by more than two years when compared to sedentary individuals. In fact, according to the Harvard School of Public Health, your life expectancy increases about two hours for every hour of regular exercise. So we should add the following to our list of benefits of being fit:

- You will look and feel younger than your chronological age.

- You will probably live longer – if you are physically fit.

Knowledge is Required for Success

Certainly, the desire to be fit and the discipline to start and stay on a fitness program are crucial. But along with desire and discipline, it is our belief that **only an in-depth understanding of weight control, nutrition and exercise will lead to long-term success**. As is true with many important and complex subjects, to achieve you need more than rules – you need a solid understanding. In this eBook we will concentrate on exercise.

We leave motivation to others. Our mission is to impart the facts, data, knowledge and the systematic approach needed for enduring physical fitness. So take the time to read what follows. The reward will last you a lifetime.

3. HOW FIT ARE YOU?

Stated or not, everyone has goals in mind when they embark on an exercise program. It could be reducing the risk of illness, losing weight, or becoming stronger. Before you begin your program, however, you should know where you stand, i.e., your current fitness level. Assessing your current level in areas such as aerobic (cardio) capacity, strength, flexibility, body-fat, and even how appropriate your nutritional practices are, will help you establish what you should emphasize in your physical fitness program and help you set goals.

Get a Medical Assessment

In our opinion, everyone should have a medical assessment, or exam, before starting a physical fitness program. The medical checkup may be as simple as a visit to a physician who is familiar with your medical history, or it may be a thorough physical exam.

Note, in all cases the physician conducting the medical exam should be made aware of and should approve the specific physical fitness program you're planning. In addition, if you have or suspect you have cardiovascular disease or other health problems, if you are obese, if you have been totally inactive, or if you are 40 or older, before embarking on a physical fitness program you should have a stress test supervised by a physician. Specific age-dependent guidelines are as follows:

Ages 20-29: For most young people in this age group a medical checkup will probably be a rather quick, basic medical exam.

Ages 30-39: The medical exam is somewhat more extensive for this age group and should include a resting EKG.

Ages 40-59: Those in this age category should proceed with still more care by having an exercising or stress-type EKG as part of their medical exam.

Ages 60 +: The medical checkup for people in this category is basically the same as for the 40-59 year olds.

To repeat, in all cases the physician conducting the medical exam should be made aware of and should approve the specific physical fitness routine you are planning. Some gyms, health clubs and fitness centers also offer a complete fitness evaluation where your aerobic capacity, strength, flexibility are body-fat percentage are determined before you sign on to a program. Besides being a good indicator of what sort of shape you are in, these tests give you a baseline you can use to judge your progress after some time on a fitness program. Alternatively, you can also get a good indication of your overall condition by taking some body measurements and performing a few simple tests as outlined in the following pages.

Aerobic-Capacity (Cardio) Self-Assessment

A good measure of aerobic capacity, or cardio-respiratory fitness, is the volume of oxygen per minute per kilogram of body weight (called VO_{2max}) a person can process during hard exercise. Higher values of VO_{2max} indicate better aerobic fitness. For example, a 25 year-old man in excellent physical condition can process about 50 milliliters of oxygen per minute per kilogram of body weight; compared to less than 20 mL/min/kg for a 70 year-old woman in poor condition.

One of the best self assessment tests for VO_{2max} is the <u>Rockport Walking Test</u>. This is a field test, not a laboratory test, and consists of walking one mile (1609 meters) as rapidly as you can. At the end of the test you record your pulse and the time required to complete the walk. You then convert the time to completion and your pulse into VO_{2max} using the formulae (on the following page). Lastly, you enter Table 3.1 (also on the next page) with your calculated VO_{2max} and determine your cardio-respiratory fitness level. There is some risk if you take the Rockport Fitness Walking Test without prior conditioning. That is why the following precautions are suggested.

1) Be sure to have a medical exam before taking the walking test.

2) If you are over 30 years old, postpone the walking test until you have been exercising regularly for at least one month.

3) You must be able to comfortably walk at least two miles before you take the walking test.

4) When you take the test, if you feel exhausted, experience shortness of breath, become dizzy or light headed, or nauseous, stop the test. Do not attempt a retest until you have exercised regularly for at least another three

months, when your fitness level should have improved.

The One-Mile (1609 meter) Walking Test

If available, walk on a school track or a measured and marked flat trail with a smooth surface. (A standard track is one-quarter mile, so walk four laps on the inside lane for the one-mile test.) You also can use a treadmill rather than a track. Although not as accurate, if need be you can walk a street course you have driven and measured. Before you start the test, warm up for several minutes with easy walking and stretching. Rest for about one minute. Then start the test. Walk as briskly as possible for one mile, but remember you'll probably walk at least 12 minutes, so don't start too fast. Pick up the pace on the last lap if you still feel strong.

When you finish the test, it's important to immediately measure your pulse. (See page 43 for recommended pulse measurement techniques.) At the conclusion of the test, you should feel slightly winded, but you should not be gasping for air. Your goal is to end the test feeling tired but not exhausted. Remember to cool down by continuing to walk slowly for a few minutes.

Gender	Age	Cardio-Respiratory Fitness Level			
		Poor	Fair	Good	Excellent
Men	20-29	33.0 - 36.4	36.5 - 42.4	42.5 - 46.4	46.5 - 52.4
	30-39	31.5 - 35.4	35.5 - 40.9	41.0 - 44.9	45.0 - 49.4
	40-49	30.2 - 33.5	33.6 - 38.9	39.0 - 43.7	43.8 - 48.0
	50-59	26.1 - 30.9	31.0 - 35.7	35.8 - 40.9	41.0 - 45.3
	60+	20.5 - 26.0	26.1 - 32.2	32.3 - 36.4	36.5 - 44.2
Women	20-29	23.6 - 28.9	29.0 - 32.9	33.0 - 36.9	37.0 - 41.0
	30-39	22.8 - 26.9	27.0 - 31.4	31.5 - 35.6	35.7 - 40.0
	40-49	21.0 - 24.4	24.5 - 28.9	29.0 - 32.8	32.9 - 36.9
	50-59	20.2 - 22.7	22.8 - 26.9	27.0 - 31.4	31.5 - 35.7
	60+	17.5 - 20.1	20.2 - 24.4	24.5 - 30.2	30.3 - 31.4

Table 3.1: VO$_{2\text{max}}$ versus Fitness Level

Calculating VO$_{2max}$: The following is undoubtedly the most difficult computation in this book, because VO$_{2max}$ is a function of so many variables: gender, weight, age, heart rate and time to complete the one-mile test walk. Although the formulae are relatively complex, we have tried to simplify the calculation as much as possible.

The formula for women is: $VO_{2max} = 133 - W - H - A - T$

The formula for men is: $VO_{2max} = 139 - W - H - A - T$

where $W = 0.077 \times$ Weight (lbs) $A = 0.39 \times$ Age
     $H = 0.157 \times$ Heart rate $T = 3.26 \times$ Time for mile

<u>Example 3.1</u>: Determine VO$_{2max}$ and the fitness level of a 29 year-old woman who weighs 10st 5lb (65.9 kilos). She finished the one-mile walking test (1609 metres) in 15 minutes and 30 seconds (which is 15.5 minutes) with a heart rate of 145 beats per minute.

The first step is to determine values for W, H, A and T.

$$W = 0.077 \times \text{Weight} = 0.077 \times 65.9 = 11.20$$

$$H = 0.157 \times \text{Heart rate} = 0.157 \times 145 \text{ beats/min} = 22.77$$

$$A = 0.39 \times \text{Age} = 0.39 \times 29 \text{ years} = 11.31$$

$$T = 3.26 \times \text{Time} = 3.26 \times 14.5 \text{ minutes} = 50.53$$

Then calculate VO$_{2max}$ using the formula for women.

$$VO_{2max} = 133 - W - H - A - T = 133 - 11.20 - 22.77 - 11.31 - 50.53 = 37.2$$

Finally, enter Table 3.1 (on page 20) for a 29 year-old woman with VO$_{2max}$ = 37.2 and find her fitness level is good – actually very good bordering on excellent.

Strength Self-Assessment

Rather than the one repetition with maximum load strength-assessment approach, we prefer the much safer anaerobic muscular strength measuring technique, where your strength is assessed by the number of repetitions you can perform with a sub-maximal load. Moreover, in the tests that follow you will use your own body weight to determine how strong you are. The standard tests are: the push-up test, the sit-up test, and the squat test. Because the sit-up test can aggravate existing lower back problems, we only recommend the press-up and squat tests. The objective in both tests is to see how many push-up and squat repetitions you can perform without stopping.

Press-up Test: For the test, men should execute the standard military push-up; i.e., your back and trunk should be rigid and straight and your weight should be supported by your arms and toes. Women should employ the familiar half push-up, supporting their weight with their arms and knees. Use Table 3.2 on the next page to assess your performance.

Squat Test: Stand about 30 cm in front of a chair. Place your feet about shoulder width apart and extend your arms parallel to the floor to your front. Bend your knees and slowly lower your body until your butt just touches the seat of the chair. (But don't sit on the chair.) Then slowly return to the standing position. Repeat as often as you can without stopping. Use Table 3.3 on the next page to assess your performance.

Gender	Age	Push-up Performance		
		Below Average	Average	Above Average
Men	20-29	15 - 24	25 - 34	35 - 44
	30-39	10 - 19	20 - 29	30 - 34
	40-49	5 - 14	15 - 24	25 - 29
	50-59	0 - 9	10 - 19	20 - 24
	60-69	0 - 4	5 - 9	10 - 15
	70+	0 - 2	3 - 5	6 - 8
Women	20-29	0 - 16	17 - 33	34 - 50
	30-39	0 - 11	12 - 24	25 - 37
	40-49	0 - 7	8 - 19	20 - 29
	50-59	0 - 5	6 - 14	15 - 23
	60+	0 - 2	3 - 5	6 - 8

Table 3.2: Strength Assessment: Push-up Performance

Gender	Age	Squat-Test Performance		
		Below Average	**Average**	**Above Average**
Men	20-29	24 - 26	27 - 29	30 - 32
	30-39	21 - 23	24 - 26	27 - 29
	40-49	18 - 20	21 - 23	24 - 26
	50-59	15 - 17	18 - 20	21 - 23
	60+	12 - 14	15 - 17	18 – 20
Women	20-29	17 - 19	21 - 23	24 - 26
	30-39	15 - 17	18 - 20	21 - 23
	40-49	12 - 14	15 - 17	18 - 20
	50-59	9 - 11	12 - 14	15 - 17
	60+	6 - 8	9 - 11	12 - 14

Table 3.3: Strength Assessment: Squat-Test Performance

Flexibility Self-Assessment

Sit & Reach Test: This is a standard test to determine hip and trunk flexibility and is often used as a measure of overall flexibility. Remember to warm up with a few gentle stretches before you start the test. To conduct the test, tape a yardstick to the floor at the 23 cm mark. Remove your shoes and sit on the floor, with your legs forward and fully extended, so that the yardstick is between and almost parallel to your extended legs. (The yardstick's zero mark should be closest to you). Locate your heels at the 23-cm mark and move your feet about 25 cm apart. Place one hand over the other and slowly stretch forward (without jerking or bouncing), and extend the tips of your fingers as far as possible along the yardstick. Repeat three times. Your score is the furthest or highest number you are able to reach. Use Table 3.4 on page 24 to assess your flexibility.

Body-Weight Self Assessment

Most people want to know what their proper or "best" body weight should be. Your weight as measured on a bathroom scale, however, can actually be misleading and certainly does not tell the whole story. The typical human body is a combination of bones, ligaments, tendons, organs, fluids, muscle and fat. When you lose or gain weight both your overall weight as well as the ratio of these components to one another changes.

Gender	Age	Sit & Reach Test Performance		
		Below Average	Average	Above Average
Men	20-29	10.0 - 13.4	13.5 - 17.0	17.1- 20.5
	30-39	9.5 - 12.9	13.0 - 16.5	16.6 -20.0
	40-49	9.0 - 12.4	12.5 - 16.0	16.1 -19.5
	50-59	8.5 - 11.9	12.0 - 15.5	15.6 - 19.0
	60+	6.0 - 9.9	10.0 - 14.0	14.1 - 18.0
Women	20-29	14.5 - 17.4	17.5 - 20.5	20.6 - 23.5
	30-39	13.5 - 16.4	16.5 - 19.5	19.6 - 22.5
	40-49	10.0 - 14.4	14.5 - 19.0	19.1 - 22.0
	50-59	10.0 - 14.4	14.5 - 17.5	17.6 - 20.5
	60+	10.0 - 13.9	14.0 - 17.0	17.1 - 20.0

Table 3.4: Flexibility Assessment: Sit & Reach Test

Exercise physiologists consider the quantity of body fat compared to total body weight a critical measure of fitness, and contend, from the standpoint of good health. Table 3.5 shows the age-adjusted fat percentage for men and women men should have no more

	Age	Underweight	Healthy	Overweight	Obese
Men	20 - 40	Less than 8 %	8 – 19 %	19 – 25 %	Over 25 %
	41 - 60	Less than 11 %	11 – 22 %	22 – 27 %	Over 27 %
	61 - 80	Less than 13 %	13 – 25 %	25 – 30 %	Over 30 %
Women	20 - 40	Less than 21 %	21 – 33 %	33 – 39 %	Over 39 %
	41 - 60	Less than 23 %	23 – 35 %	35 – 40 %	Over 40 %
	61 - 80	Less than 24 %	24 – 36 %	36 – 42 %	Over 42 %

Table 3.5: Age-Adjusted Body Fat Percentage for Men & Women*

* Source: Gallagher et al., Am J Clin Nut 2000; 72:694-701

Percent body fat is estimated in a number of ways. The most accurate, used in many research laboratories, involves underwater or hydrostatic weighing to determine body density from which the percentage of body fat can be computed. The body fat percentage (and fitness) of many professional athletes is measured by under-water weighing. Lately, obesity researchers have started to use bioelectrical impedance testing and magnetic resonance imaging to measure body fat. None of these methods, however, are practical for personal use, and more convenient means have been devised whereby body fat can be estimated. For more information and tables to determine body fat percentage see Professional Weight Control for Men and Professional Weight Control for Women published by NoPaperPress. Both books have age-related body fat percentages and waist sizes for men and women.

More recently, physicians and some scientists use a parameter called the Body Mass Index, or BMI, to determine if a person is overweight. The BMI takes into account both a person's weight and height and is calculated by dividing a person's weight in kilograms by their height in meters squared. Scientists categorize a man or woman's weight profile (Table 3.7) as a function of BMI. For readers living in the UK, Table 3.6 allows the determination of the BMI using body weight in stones and height in centimeters.

Weight (st.)	- Height (cm.) -									
	155	160	165	170	175	180	185	190	195	200
7	18.5									
8	21.2	19.9	18.7							
9	23.8	22.4	21.0	19.8	18.7					
10	26.5	24.8	23.4	22.0	20.8	19.6	18.6			
11	29.1	27.3	25.7	24.2	22.8	21.6	20.4	19.4	18.4	
12	31.8	29.8	28.0	26.4	24.9	23.6	22.3	21.1	20.1	19.1
13	34.4	32.3	30.4	28.6	27.0	25.5	24.2	22.9	21.7	20.7
14	37.1	34.8	32.7	30.8	29.1	27.5	26.0	24.7	23.4	22.3
15	39.7	37.3	35.0	33.0	31.2	29.4	27.9	26.4	25.1	23.9
16	42.4	39.8	37.4	35.2	33.2	31.4	29.7	28.2	26.8	25.4
17	45.0	42.2	39.7	37.4	35.3	33.4	31.6	30.0	28.4	27.0
18	47.7	44.7	42.0	39.6	37.4	35.3	33.4	31.7	30.1	28.6
20				44.0	39.5	39.3	39.0	35.2	33.5	31.8
22						43.2	40.9	38.8	36.8	35.0

Table 3.6: Body Mass Index (BMI) vs Height & Weight

BMI	Weight Profile
18.5 or less	Underweight
18.6 to 24.9	Normal
25.0 to 29.9	Overweight
30.0 to 39.9	Obese
40 or more	Extremely Obese

Table 3.7: Body Weight Profile

A more convenient way to use BMI is the New BMI-Based Weight vs. Height shown in Table 3.8, where the underweight category corresponds to BMI = 18.5 or less, normal BMI = 18.6 to 24.9, overweight BMI = 25.0 to 29.9, obese is BMI = 30.0 to 39.9 and extremely obese is BMI = 40 or more.

Height (cm)	Under (kg)	Normal (kg)	Over (kg)	Obese (kg)	Very Obese
150	41 or less	42 – 56	57 – 67	68 – 90	> 91
153	43 or less	44 – 58	59 – 70	71 – 93	> 94
156	45 or less	46 – 61	62 – 73	74 – 97	> 98
159	47 or less	48 – 63	64 – 76	77 – 101	> 102
162	49 or less	50 – 65	66 – 79	80 – 105	> 106
165	50 or less	51 – 68	69 – 81	82 – 109	> 110
168	52 or less	53 – 70	71 – 84	85 – 113	> 114
171	54 or less	55 – 73	74 – 87	88 – 117	> 118
174	56 or less	57 – 75	76 – 90	91 – 121	> 122
177	58 or less	59 – 78	79 – 94	95 – 125	> 126
180	60 or less	61 – 81	82 – 97	98 – 129	> 130
183	62 or less	63 – 83	84 – 100	101 – 134	> 135
186	64 or less	65 – 86	87 – 103	104 – 138	> 139
189	**140 or less**	67 – 89	90 – 107	108 – 143	> 144

Table 3.8: BMI-Based Weight vs. Height

Weight Assessment Example

<u>Example 3.2</u>: Consider a man who is 185 cm tall and weighs 15 stone (95.5 kg) and who has a 112 cm waist and his hip measures 91cm. Determine his "best weight range" using two methods: a) BMI, Tables 3.6 and 3.7, b) Table 3.8, "BMI-Based Weight Range vs. Height."

a) <u>BMI Method</u>: Table 3.6 (on page 25 shows that at 185 cm and 15 stone his BMI = 27.9 and that he is overweight. Table 3.7 also indicates that to get to the normal range, which requires a BMI of at most 24.9, he would have get his weight down to approximately 13 stone.

b) <u>BMI-Based Weight Range vs. Height Table</u>: From Table 3.8 (on page 26, we note that for a 185 cm man anything over 85 kg is considered overweight, and that he would have to weigh between 64 and 84 kg to be deemed "normal weight."

Waist-to-Hip Ratio: Another very important weight-profile parameter is your waist-to-hip ratio. Health risks for heart attack and stroke increase considerably for men that have a waist to hip ratio greater than 1.0, and for women that have a waist to hip ratio greater than 0.8.

To calculate your ratio, measure your waist size (at its narrowest circumference) and divide it by your hip size (at the widest section). For example, a man with a 111-cm waist and 91-cm hip would have a waist to hip ratio of 111/91 = 1.2, and would have an increased risk for a heart attack or stroke.

Now Set Goals

To this point, in Chapter 1 we defined the problem; in Chapter 2 we outlined a "fitness prescription," and in Chapter 3 we briefly set forth techniques you can use to assess your aerobic capacity, your strength, your flexibility and

your body weight, i.e., your current total fitness level. Now it's time to review your fitness-self-assessment test results and set some broad personal fitness goals, such improving your aerobic capacity. You're not quite ready to construct a total program. That will have to wait until you read the in-depth exercise chapter that follows.

4. EXERCISE FOR HEALTH

Many of us exist largely through mental efforts - by our wits and skill. All the advances of modern technology – from washing machines to automobiles to computers – have made life easier, or at least physically much less demanding. For most people, the common tasks of living and working no longer provide enough exercise to develop and maintain cardiovascular and respiratory fitness and good muscle tone. With any luck we can go for weeks without working up a good sweat or drawing a deep breath! Our bodies, however, are virtually identical to that of primitive humans who survived through physical efforts – by strength and stamina.

In fact, the bodies we inherited are just not built to be immobile and passive. The sad fact, however, is that after years of education and information programs by government agencies, medical associations and insurance companies relatively few Americans engage in regular planned exercise – despite the reality that we need to be active to keep our systems working efficiently and to rid ourselves of emotional tension.

There are two ways to become more physically active: 1) Increase the physical activity in your daily life; and 2) Start on a regular exercise program. Better still would be a combination of both.

Be More Active Every Day

Before we address exercise programs, here are some ways you can increase physical activity in your daily routine:

1. Change your attitude toward the occasional "bothersome" physical tasks that you encounter in daily living. Consider anytime you have to lift, bend, reach, walk as an opportunity to burn additional calories and as an extension of your formal workout.

2. Look for opportunities to walk, such as walking up stairs (two at a time if you can) rather than using an elevator, walking to a local store rather than driving, walking the course if you play golf, and mowing your lawn. At work stand up and stretch two or three times a day, read standing up, etcetera.

3. Engage in leisure activities such as dancing, bowling and gardening more often. They can be enjoyable and provide added exercise.

Each of these daily activities taken alone may not seem like much, but done every day for many years they can add up to a substantial number of extra calories burned.

Energy Used For Different Activities

Table 4.1 (on the next page) shows the number of calories burned per hour for various activities. Although the data in the table are from reliable sources, you may find that some of the values are slightly different than those in other books. There are several reasons for this. First, the intensity of the activity being measured may actually vary (for instance handball can be played at many different levels – with a different number of calories burned at each level). Then the calories burned by same-weight individuals engaged in the same activity does vary somewhat; and finally measurement techniques and data collection accuracy vary slightly from laboratory to laboratory. The best one can do, therefore, is arrive at an average from the available data, which often requires judgment and compromise. More important, notice that the calories expended for a given activity depends on your weight. Good news: **For any activity, the more you weigh the more calories you burn!**

Calories Burned Example

Example 4.1: Determine the number of calories burned by a 13st 7lb man (or woman) who walks 11 kilometres in two hours.

First calculate the person's walking speed = 11 km / 2 hours = 5.5 km/hr. Because 13st 7lb is not listed in Table 4.1 (on the next page), we use the neighboring value of 14 st. Then from Table 4.1 find that walking at 5.5 km/hr, a person weighing 14 stone burns 388 kcalories per hour. In two hours, therefore, a person weighing 14 stone would burn, 2 x 388 = 776 kcalories.

But from this we must subtract the number of calories a 14 stone person would have used anyway if, instead of walking, he or she just sat for the two hours. From Table 4.1 this amounts to 114 kcalories per hour, or 228 kcalories in two hours. Then the net energy a 14 stone person would expend walking (over and above just sitting) totals 776 – 228 = 548 kcalories. However, the individual in this example weighs 13st 7lb (13.5 stone) and would expend proportionately fewer calories than a person that weighs 14 stone, and therefore would burn: 548 x 13.5 / 14 = 528 kcalories

Activity	Weight (Stone)								
	9	10	11	12	13	14	16	18	20
Aerobics (dance)	516	573	630	687	745	802	917	1031	1146
Basketball	401	445	490	534	579	623	712	801	890
Bicycling (13 mph)	458	508	559	610	661	712	814	915	1017
Cycling (stationary)	401	445	490	534	579	623	712	801	890
Cricket	284	315	347	378	410	441	504	567	630
Dancing (ballroom)	262	292	321	350	379	408	466	525	583
Golf (pulling cart)	284	315	347	378	410	441	504	567	630
Golf (riding cart)	199	222	244	266	288	310	354	399	443
Handball	384	426	469	512	554	597	682	768	853
Hiking	336	373	411	448	486	523	598	672	747
Hockey (ice/field)	451	502	552	602	652	702	802	903	1003
Horseback riding	226	251	276	301	326	351	401	451	501
Jogging	714	793	873	952	1032	1111	1270	1428	1587
Mowing lawn	314	349	384	419	454	489	559	629	699
Raking leaves	345	383	421	459	498	536	613	689	766
Rowing (moderate)	399	443	488	532	577	621	710	798	887
Sitting	73	82	90	98	106	114	130	147	163
Skating	399	443	488	532	577	621	710	798	887
Skiing (+ country)	457	508	559	609	660	711	813	914	1016
Skiing (downhill)	347	385	424	462	501	539	616	693	770
Skipping rope	480	533	587	640	694	747	854	960	1067
Soccer (football)	431	479	526	574	622	670	766	861	957
Softball	284	315	347	378	410	441	504	567	630
Squash	384	426	469	512	554	597	682	768	853
Swimming laps	462	513	565	616	668	719	822	924	1027
Tennis (singles)	336	373	411	448	486	523	598	672	747
Tennis (doubles)	255	283	311	339	368	396	453	509	566
Walking (4.8 kph)	204	227	249	272	294	317	362	408	453
Walking (5.5 kph)	249	277	305	333	360	388	443	499	554
Walking (6.5 kph)	317	353	387	423	458	493	563	634	704

Table 4.1: Energy Expended (kcal per hour) for Different Activities

Types of Exercise

Simply stated there are **three basic types of exercise: aerobic, stretching, and strengthening**.

1) **Aerobic exercises** (also called "cardio") condition your cardiovascular system. Aerobic exercises, such as jogging, swimming, cycling, brisk walking, skipping rope, jogging in place, and many others, are typically deep breathing and continuous, with rhythmic and repetitive contractions of your large muscle groups. Most aerobic exercises have one thing in common: they make you work hard and require you to process a great deal of oxygen.

   In fact, aerobic is a word derived from the Greek, meaning "with oxygen." Aerobic activities require oxygen for the production of energy. The main goal of an aerobic exercise program is to increase the rate which your body can process oxygen, i.e., increase VO_{2max}. A well-conditioned person with efficient lungs and a strong heart can pump large volumes of blood, can breathe large volumes of air, and via the blood circulatory system effectively transport the oxygen in the air they breathe to all parts of their body.

   During aerobic exercise, the large muscles of the body continuously flood the heart with a great deal of blood; the heart beats faster; blood flow rate increases; and the lungs transport large quantities of oxygen to the blood. Regular exercise of this type "trains" the heart to pump more blood with less effort. Aerobic exercise improves the circulatory system by developing more elastic arteries and by creating peripheral or extra blood paths to the heart; and aerobic exercise strengthens the muscles of respiration increasing the volume of oxygen that can be processed within a given time. Done regularly, aerobic exercises improve stamina and endurance, and most importantly promote what should be your central exercise goal - cardiovascular fitness. For if your cardiovascular system is not in shape, you're not in shape - no matter how many push-ups or crunches you can do! In net, aerobic exercises develop a powerful heart, an effective circulatory system and efficient lungs.

   Aerobic exercises can be further subdivided according to how strenuous they are and how well they condition the heart and lungs. (Note, there are exercises other than those shown that could be included in the groupings that follow.)

Group A: Bicycling, Cross-country skiing, Dancing (aerobic), Hiking in rugged terrain, Ice Hockey, Jogging, Jogging in place, Rowing, Skipping rope, Stair climbing, and Stationary cycling.

Group B: Basketball, Field Hockey, Calisthenics, Handball, Racquetball, Skiing (downhill), Soccer, Squash, Tennis (singles), Volleyball, and Walking (briskly).

Group C: Badminton, Baseball, Bowling, Croquet, Dancing, Gardening, Golf (carrying or pulling clubs), Horseback riding, Housework, Ping-pong, Shuffleboard, Softball, Tennis (doubles) and Walking (moderate to leisurely).

The vigorous exercises in Group A are intended for those already in good condition who want to further strengthen their heart and lungs and improve their aerobic capacity. The moderate exercises in Group B are not as demanding as those in Group A, but they are nevertheless good choices and can condition your heart and lungs. The exercises in Group C are actually not aerobic because they are either low intensity or not continuous, or both, but they still can be beneficial in that they improve muscle tone and coordination, relieve tension and burn some calories. (Note that some exercises in one group if done vigorously could easily be as demanding as those in the next higher grouping. For example, a very intense game of squash could move it from the Group B to the Group A category.)

As a final point, please note that the exercise portion of *Exercise for Better Health* is aimed at the beginner who wants to improve his or her fitness level and general health, and someone who has already attained some degree of fitness but wants to learn more and go on to the next level. It is not intended for individuals who want to be highly-conditioned athletes and so topics such as interval, tempo and uphill training methods are not covered. (On the other hand, people at all fitness levels will find the information in *Total Fitness - U.S. Edition* Chapter 5 "Nutrition Basics" and Chapter 6 "Weight Control" extremely valuable.)

2) **Stretching-type exercises** such as yoga, tai chi, Pilates and to a lesser extent calisthenics can improve your flexibility – and some of the exercises can make you somewhat stronger.

As you age you inevitably start to loose flexibility. Your gait becomes stiffer; you can't stand quite as upright as you used to; it becomes tougher to bend over; and you have difficulty turning your neck. Regardless of your age, however, stretching can make you more flexible, less injury prone, and can reduce the pain and discomfort associated with tight muscles and shortened tendons. Realize, however, that stretching exercises do not condition your heart and lungs. Stretching exercises are fine as long as they are performed in addition to rather than in place of an aerobic exercise.

Most experts do recommend stretching before and after aerobic and strength routines. However, never stretch cold muscles and always do some form of warm up prior to stretching. Stretch slowly and hold gently. You should stretch to the point of feeling a mild pull, but you should never feel pain. And when you stretch – do not bounce.

3) **Muscle building and strengthening exercises,** e.g., weight lifting, use of the machines found in fitness centers and isometrics.

Once more, as you age you loose muscle mass, your bone density decreases and you lose strength. Exercises like weight lifting strengthen your muscles, bones and joints. Strengthening exercises also reduce your risk of developing osteoporosis, a severe bone-loss disease, which can lead to easily fractured bones and all the complications that often follow. Strong muscles not only allow you to lift a sleepy four-year old out of a car without difficulty and lug groceries up to a second floor apartment, but as with increased flexibility, strong muscles also make you less injury prone. **Strengthening exercises are beneficial and should be a part of your fitness routine, but again they should be performed in addition to an aerobic exercise** because alone they cannot condition your heart and lungs.

Select the Correct Exercise for You

Selecting the right fitness exercise is the key to a successful conditioning program. You should try to pick an activity (or activities) you will enjoy. Factors to consider in choosing your activity are: your medical condition, your age, your fitness level, your exercise goals, your daily and overall schedule, exercise outdoors or indoors, exercise alone or with others, and how much money you are prepared to spend. You may decide to concentrate on one activity such as squash, or you may choose to walk briskly some days and lift weights on other days. Incidentally, three to five days of a vigorous aerobic exercise plus two days of either strength or flexibility exercises per week is a good combination. Whatever you settle on make sure it is an activity (or activities) that can be done regularly and that you enjoy.

Your Medical Condition: If you have a medical condition such as a heart problem, diabetes, osteoporosis, etcetera, or if you are a female who is pregnant or breast-feeding, you should proceed with caution, and be sure to talk to your doctor before you start any exercise activity.

Your Age: The age-dependent guidelines for how to proceed are as follows:

Ages 20-29: Assuming a clean bill of health from a medical exam, young men and women – unless badly overweight – can usually start an exercise program immediately.

Ages 30-39: The precautions here are the same as for the 20-29 year-old age group except that the medical checkup should also include a resting EKG.

Ages 40-59: Those in this age category should proceed with still more care by having an exercising or stress-type EKG as part of their medical exam.

Ages 60-up: The medical checkup is the same as for the 40-59 year old group. (Unless one has been physically active for a number of years, most physicians feel that at this age exercise should be limited to walking and moderate flexibility and/or strengthening exercises to improve muscle tone.)

Your Fitness Level: If you have been inactive for some time, rather than starting with one of the more strenuous exercises, **beginners of all ages should initially confine themselves to walking** until they can easily walk about 3½ km at a brisk pace. When you reach this stage more strenuous exercises can be attempted if desired. Furthermore, some sports medicine physicians contend that **if you are badly overweight you should limit your exercise to walking** until you have lost weight to the point where you are less than 25 percent overweight. For example, a 185 cm tall man who weighs 18 stone 8 pounds, from Table 3.6 (on page 28), has a best weight of about 13 stone (182 lbs). Twenty-five percent of 182 lbs is 46 lbs. Therefore, he should limit his exercise to walking until he has reduced his weight to less than (182 + 46), or about 16st 4lb.

Your Exercise Goals: If you want to strengthen your heart and lungs, improve your aerobic capacity and burn a lot of calories select an aerobic activity from Group A or B. If you want to improve your flexibility select a stretching type exercise. And if you want to become physically stronger choose one of the strength-building exercises.

Your Schedule: Only you know what the demands on your time from work, family and your social life are. What is the best time of day for you? Which days of the week best fit your schedule? Of course, you must be open to rearranging your priorities to fit exercise into your daily life.

Outdoors or Indoors: If you decide to exercise outdoors you should also have an alternate indoor activity, an activity you can fall back on in bad weather. For example, if you choose to jog outside early in the morning before work, you may want to purchase a treadmill for use at home on days when it is either too hot, too cold or the weather is bad.

Alone or with Others: On the plus side, an exercise partner can make exercise more enjoyable and can help you get going and keep going on days when you might otherwise quit. On the other hand, a partner probably means that you have the schedules of two busy people to contend with and plan around, which can at times actually hinder your workout.

How Much Are You Prepared to Spend: For many activities, you will need little or no special equipment. For instance, walking outside only requires comfortable shoes; whereas, joining and working out at a fitness center can be relatively expensive.

Aerobic Exercise: How Hard?

Because cardiovascular fitness should be your prime concern, **the central part of your exercise program should be an aerobic (or cardio) exercise done regularly**. Additional stretching and strengthening exercises should be included as time allows – but never to the exclusion of the aerobic portion of your program.

An aerobic exercise program should be vigorous enough to condition the cardiovascular system but not so strenuous as to exceed safe limits. Some experts define safe as an exercise pace that is "comfortable." What they mean is that if, for instance, you are jogging or walking briskly you should be able to converse comfortably with a partner. They add that you should be breathing and feeling normally within ten minutes after you stop exercising. If not you are exercising too vigorously. Other signs that you are pushing too hard include difficulty breathing, feeling faint, or feeling weak – during or after exercising. If you experience any of these symptoms, you are exercising too intensely and you should cut back.

Others prefer a more quantitative definition. They refer to the beneficial yet safe exercise region as the "Target Training Zone," or TTZ, which is determined by monitoring your pulse. The idea is to raise your pulse through exercise to a specific range (the target training zone) and hold it there for an extended period to obtain a cardiovascular benefit. On this concept rests the so-called heart-rated theory of exercise, which relies on heart rate (or pulse) to establish the proper exercise intensity.

Aerobic Exercise: Target-Training Zone

The **Target-Training Zone (TTZ) is a measure of aerobic exercise intensity**. Use the following procedure to calculate your individual target-training zone:

1) Calculate your **Maximum heart rate** = 220 – Age in years. (Your maximum heart rate is the fastest your heart can beat, and you definitely must exercise well below this level.)

2) Compute your **Maximum heart rate reserve** = Maximum heart rate minus your resting pulse.

3) Lastly, calculate your **TTZ** pulse = (Maximum heart rate reserve multiplied by Exercise intensity level) + Resting pulse.

If you would rather not do the mathematics, you may determine your TTZ from Tables 4.2 and 4.3 (on pages 37 and 38). But before that, you need to determine the exercise intensity level that is right for you.

Aerobic Exercise: Intensity Guidelines

Many exercise physiologists recommend the following guidelines:

1. <u>Low Exercise-Intensity Level:</u> This intensity level should be used by anyone over 50 years old, and by those starting a physical fitness program after many years of inactivity regardless of their age. People in this classification should begin exercising at 40 to 50% of their TTZ.

2. <u>Moderate Exercise-Intensity Level:</u> This applies to moderately active people who are under 50 years old and who, for example, have been

walking two or three miles per day regularly. These men and women may begin exercising at 50 to 65% of their TTZ.

3. <u>High Exercise-Intensity Level:</u> This level applies to very active, well-trained, fit people under 50 years old. These individuals may exercise at 65 to 80% of their TTZ.

Age	Resting Pulse	Exercise Intensity (%)				
		40	50	60	70	80
	50	110	125	140	155	170
20	60	116	130	144	158	172
	70	122	135	148	161	174
	80	128	140	140	164	176
	50	108	123	137	152	166
25	60	114	128	141	155	168
	70	120	133	145	158	170
	80	126	138	149	161	172
	50	106	120	134	148	162
30	60	112	125	138	151	164
	70	118	130	142	154	166
	80	124	135	146	157	168
	50	104	118	131	145	158
35	60	110	123	135	148	160
	70	116	128	139	151	162
	80	122	133	143	154	164
	50	102	115	128	141	154
40	60	108	120	132	144	156
	70	114	125	136	147	158
	80	120	130	140	150	160

Table 4.2: Target-Training Zone: Ages 20 to 40 years

Age	Resting Pulse	Exercise Intensity (%)				
		40	50	60	70	80
45	50	100	113	125	138	150
	60	106	118	129	141	152
	70	112	123	133	144	154
	80	118	128	137	147	156
50	50	98	110	122	134	146
	60	104	115	126	137	148
	70	110	120	130	140	150
	80	116	125	134	143	152
55	50	96	108	119	131	142
	60	102	113	123	134	144
	70	108	118	127	137	146
	80	114	123	131	140	148
60	50	94	105	116	127	138
	60	100	110	120	130	140
	70	106	115	124	133	142
	80	112	120	128	136	144
65	50	92	103	113	124	134
	60	98	108	117	127	136
	70	104	113	121	130	138
	80	110	118	125	133	140

Table 4.3: Target-Training Zone: Ages 45 to 65 years

If you do use the target-training zone approach, your pulse becomes your exercise guide. In addition, after a couple of months of aerobic exercise a sure indication that you are rounding into shape, making progress, is that your resting pulse slows down somewhat – especially if it was relatively fast at the start. This is because well-conditioned strengthened hearts are more efficient and so beat more slowly at rest. Trained athletes often have a resting pulse of 50 beats per minute or lower, whereas the "average" pulse is 72 to 76 for untrained men and 75 to 80 for untrained women. Furthermore, understand that as you become more physically fit you will have to exercise more vigorously to get your exercising pulse rate into your target-training zone.

Target-Training Zone Example

Example 4.2:   Determine the target-training zone (TTZ) for a 40-year old relatively inactive man with a resting pulse of 70, whose physician has approved his intention to start an aerobic exercise program.

Because he is relatively inactive but also relatively young, following the exercise-intensity level guidelines outlined earlier, he determines that he may start his exercise program at about 50 percent of his maximum heart rate reserve. He determines his (TTZ) as follows:

Maximum heart rate = 220 – Age in years = 220 - 40 = 180

Maximum heart rate reserve = Maximum heart rate – Resting pulse
= 180 – 70 = 110

TTZ = (Maximum heart rate reserve multiplied by Exercise intensity level) + Resting pulse = (110 x 0.50) + 70 = 125 beats per minute.

(Note, the exercise-intensity level was converted from 50 % to the decimal equivalent 0.50.)

Alternatively, the 40-year old man could have used Table 4.2, where first he would search the far left side of the table and locate his age (40). Then from the four possible resting pulse selections he would choose (70); finally he would run his finger horizontally (to the right) until he intersects the vertical column headed by the 50 percent exercise intensity level where he would find his TTZ of 125 beats per minute. Because it is difficult to get an exact pulse during or immediately after exercising and this is not an exact science, he should convert his calculated TTZ into a TTZ range. In this case, for a 50 percent exercise intensity level his TTZ range would be about 122 to 128 beats per minute.

When you cannot find your exact combination of age, resting pulse and exercise intensity level in tables 4.2 and 4.3, an estimating technique called interpolation[1] can be used to calculate your TTZ – although it would probably be easier for you to just use the formulae and procedure shown on page 36 and the mathematical procedure illustrated in Example 4.2.

Aerobic Exercise: Duration & Frequency

The American College of Sports Medicine recommends that an exercise heart rate of 60 to 90 percent of your maximum heart rate should be maintained for

---

1. A description of the mathematical procedure called interpolation is beyond the scope of this book.

about 30 to 45 minutes three to five days per week to become reasonably fit. They also stated, "For most people exercising at the lower end of their heart rate range for a longer time is better than exercising at the higher end of the range for a shorter time." The United States Surgeon General recommends that people accumulate 30 minutes of moderate activity on most, if not all, days of the week. More recently, the U.S. Institute of Medicine suggested 60 minutes of moderate exercise every day. To confuse matters even more, many exercise physiologists favor the following exercise schedule:

- <u>Low Exercise-Intensity Level</u> (40 to 50% of maximum heart rate reserve): People in this category (because of their age or lack of fitness) should work up to exercising 60 minutes per day at least five days per week. Despite the low intensity exercise level participants should achieve what exercise physiologists feel is an acceptable – albeit minimum – level of fitness.

- <u>Moderate Exercise-Intensity Level</u> (50 to 65% of maximum heart rate reserve): Men and women at this level should build up to 45 minutes of exercise per day at least five days per week to achieve a minimum fitness level.

- <u>High Exercise-Intensity Level</u> (65 to 80% of maximum heart rate reserve): In this category, individuals should work up to 30 minutes of exercise per day at least five days per week for a minimally acceptable fitness level.

As you can see, in general if you exercise at the lower exercise intensity levels your workout should last longer. Moreover, the longer and more frequently you exercise the greater your fitness reward. How fit you become is really a matter of your age, your genes, how fit you think you should be – and how hard you are willing to work. But don't overdo it! Again, it is worth repeating, everyone should have medical clearance before beginning any exercise program.

Aerobic Exercise: Typical Workout

First, do not smoke before you exercise (or after for that matter); do not eat for two hours before you start exercising, and refrain from drinking any alcohol for four hours prior to beginning your exercise routine. A classic aerobic exercise routine consists of a warm up, your main exercise, and a cool down.

- Start with a three to seven minute warm up. Three minutes of stretching is sufficient if you are going to engage in a low intensity Group C exercise such as badminton; whereas a longer seven-minute warm up is better preparation for a high intensity Group A aerobic exercises such as jogging, cycling or stair climbing.

- Then move on to 30 to 60 minutes of your main aerobic exercise.

- Finish with a three to seven minute cool down period. Once more, if you are finishing a low-intensity exercise three minutes is enough. After a moderate or high-intensity aerobic exercise a seven minute cool down is more appropriate.

Warm up: Going from a resting state to a moderate or high-intensity exercise is a large jump. The warm up period gives your body time to bridge the gap and get ready for the more strenuous exercise that follows. Tension in your muscles and nerves is released; your large-frame muscles, ligaments and joints are stretched and put through their full range of motion; and your arteries and capillaries start to dilate as your heart beats faster and your blood-flow rate increases.

Begin your warm up by walking slowly and gradually increase your pace as you approach the end of the warm up period. Next stretch. **Never stretch cold muscles**. Many stretches are based on yoga, where you start with good posture and then use your body weight to stretch your tissues. The following is a list of stretching exercises for your arms, neck, back and legs that are especially suited for warm up and cool down periods. Stretches (c) through (g) are illustrated in Figure 4.1, on page 43. (Some of these stretches can be done toward the end of the walking segment of your warm-up.) Perform the stretches as described.

a) <u>Neck Swivel</u>: From a standing position, with your arms hanging loosely, rotate your head about your neck, five times clockwise, then five times counter clockwise.

b) <u>Shoulder Roll</u>: While standing, with your arms hanging loosely at your side rotate your shoulders first in a forward motion, then backwards. Repeat five times.

c) <u>Arm Pumping</u>: Again, from a standing position, raise your elbows to shoulder height. Pull your elbows and arms slowly rearward as you thrust your chest forward. Repeat five times.

d) <u>Side to side Stretch</u>: From a standing position, raise both hands over your head. Bend slowly from side to side. Repeat five times.

e) <u>Toe Touch</u>: Sit along a bench and place your right leg on the bench. Position your left leg on the floor. Lean forward and try to touch your right toe until feel a stretch behind your right knee and calf. Do not bounce. Hold for a count of ten. Repeat with left leg raised. (This stretch can also be done from a standing position by placing a leg on a chair.)

f) <u>Wall Push to Stretch Calves</u>: Stand about two feet from a wall. Then as you extend your arms forward lean into the wall. Keep both heels flat on the floor. Do not bounce. Hold this position for a count of ten.

g) <u>Quad Stretch</u>: Balance yourself by placing your left hand on a wall. Bend your right leg and move your right heel toward your rear end. Grab your right foot with your right hand. Pull very gently. You should feel mild pressure in your right quad (the front of your right thigh). Do not bounce. Hold for a count of ten. Repeat for the left leg.

Do not feel limited to the following stretching exercises. There are many, many other good stretches available (too many to discuss here) that you might prefer.

If your main activity is a low-intensity exercise, you can conclude your warm up after stretching out. If you are going on to a moderate or high-intensity aerobic exercise, after stretching start your main aerobic exercise but at a relatively lower level. Over the next few minutes gradually increase the intensity so that your pulse approaches your target training zone. For instance, if you are a jogger you might warm up as follows: Start by walking slowly but steadily walk faster. After approximately five minutes stop and do two minutes of stretching. In theory, your warm up is over, but begin the main portion of your exercise by walking much faster, transition to a slow jog, then jog somewhat faster, and so on until, after about five minutes you have reached your regular jogging pace.

Main Exercise: Now you can begin your aerobic exercise of choice in earnest, stopping only to see that your pulse is in your target-training zone. If not, adjust your exercise level, exerting more or less effort. (Eventually, you will be able to sense that you are exercising at the correct intensity level and need only monitor your pulse occasionally.)

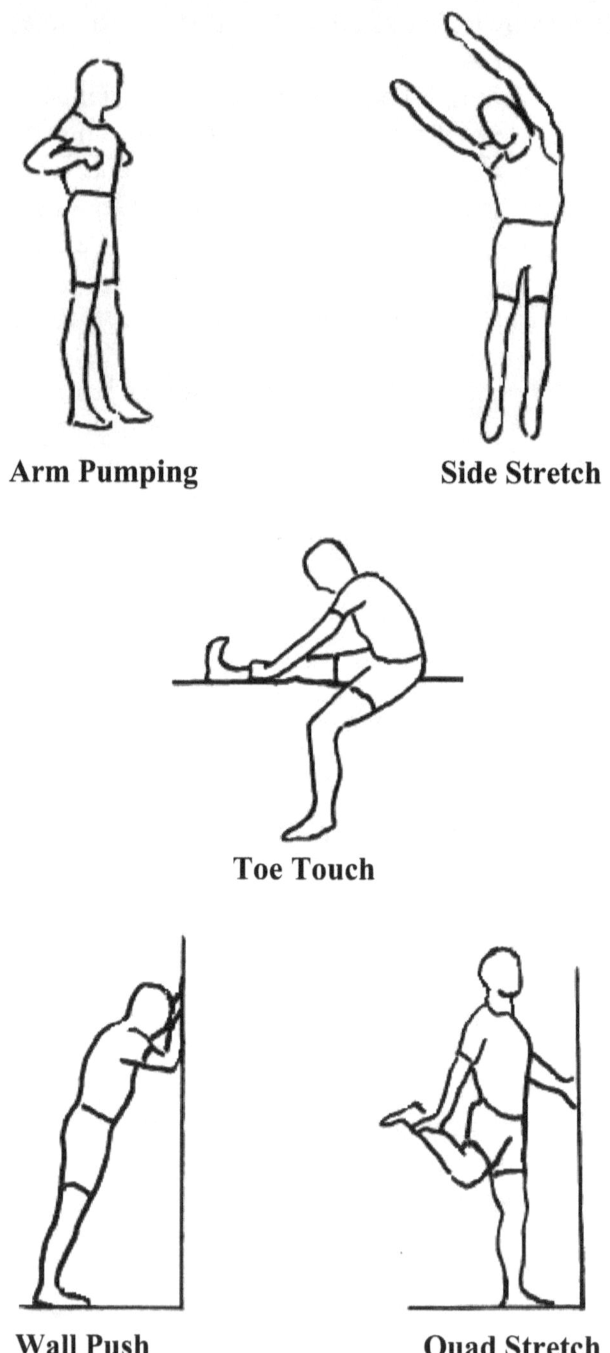

Figure 4.1: Stretching Exercises (c) to (g)

Cool Down: A five to seven-minute cooling off period should follow an aerobic workout. During cool down keep moving, decrease your activity level slowly. End your workout with leg stretches such as toe touches, a wall push and a quad stretch.

Aerobic Exercise: Pulse Measurement

In order to monitor the intensity of exercise, you should occasionally stop during your workout and take your pulse immediately. This is because your pulse will fall quickly once you stop exercising. The trick is to find your pulse within a couple of seconds and then start counting.

Quickly place the tips of two fingers on one of the two carotid arteries in your neck. (Your carotid arteries are located on either side of your throat.) Count the beats for ten seconds and multiply by six. For example, if you count 20 beats in ten seconds then your pulse would be 120 beats per minute.

You are doing fine if your pulse is within your TTZ range. If your pulse is too slow, exercise somewhat harder; if your pulse is fast, exercise easier. Again, after you have exercised for some time you will be able to feel that you are exerting the correct amount of effort and need only check your exercising pulse about once a week.

(Note: The best way to find your resting pulse is to measure it immediately upon rising in the morning. Use the average over three days for the truest result.)

Aerobic Exercise: Monitoring Devices

The following are some other techniques and equipment you can use to measure and monitor the quality of your exercise regime.

Watch Monitor: Worn on your wrist these devices measure your exercising pulse and so much more. They are sold by Fitbit, Garmin, Apple, Samsung, etc.

Pedometer: Fastened to your belt or waistband, pedometers count steps, and once you determine your stride length a pedometer can also be used to gauge distance. Pedometers are relatively inexpensive. A Smart phone App can also be used. In weight-loss programs, people are advised to accumulate at least 10,000 steps a day (which is equivalent to walking about five miles).

G.P.S. Monitor: By determining your location, a Global Positioning System sensor can measure your speed, distance and pace during a workout.

<u>Power Meter:</u> Some cyclists use power meters to record power output, pedal revolutions, speed, time and distance. Most meters allow the data to be uploaded to a computer – but the meters can be expensive.

Aerobic Exercise: A Walking Program

If your goal is to improve your general health and fitness, walking is a wonderful exercise. It's an exercise that you can do anywhere, that you can do outdoors or indoors, that requires no special equipment other than a good comfortable pair of walking shoes, and that you can do well into your old age. Walking does have a downside. Because it is a relatively low-intensity exercise, to get a good workout you have to spend more time walking compared to most high-intensity exercises.

If you are more than 50 years old, or have been sedentary for some time, it is best to start with a walking program that slowly but surely builds in intensity. If you walk hard enough, long enough and often enough, a walking workout can make you fit. A ten-week <u>beginner's routine</u> is shown in Table 4.4 on the following page.

The first session in week 1 starts with approximately three minutes of walking at an easy pace of about 4 km/hr. Continue your warm up with two minutes of stretching. (See the stretching exercises described on pages 47 and 48.) Then start walking more briskly, about 6 km/hr, but you should check your pulse and increase or decrease this to get your heart rate into a TTZ corresponding to about a 50 percent intensity level. After eight minutes, start your cool down by reducing your walking speed again to about 4 km/hr for three minutes. Conclude your session by doing about two minutes of stretching. The total workout time in week 1 is 18 minutes per session. The only part that changes in succeeding weeks (2 through 10), is the brisk walking portion of the workout continually increases from 8 minutes in week 1 to 30 minutes in week 10.

Week	Warm up Walking Minutes	Warm up Stretching (Minutes)	Brisk Walking Minutes	Cool Down Walking Minutes	Cool Down Stretching (Minutes)	Total Minutes per Session
1	3	2	8	3	2	18
2	3	2	10	3	2	20
3	3	2	12	3	2	22
4	3	2	14	3	2	24
5	3	2	16	3	2	26
6	3	2	18	3	2	28
7	3	2	20	3	2	30
8	3	2	23	3	2	33
9	3	2	26	3	2	36
10	3	2	30	3	2	40

Table 4.4: Walking Program for Beginners

Walk at least three days a week for ten weeks. If you find a week particularly tiring, backup to the previous week (or repeat the week) before continuing with the program. This is not a contest; you do not have to finish the program in ten weeks. Once you complete the ten-week program you can either stay on a walking routine, or go on to one of the more strenuous aerobic exercises.

If you decide to become a walker and want to improve, first go from walking three days per week to five days per week – at the same TTZ. To improve further gradually increase your total workout time from 40 to 60 minutes. To improve even more, gradually increase your walking speed, and TTZ, so that your exercise intensity level approaches 60 percent. Another good way to increase the intensity of your walking workout is to include some hills in your route. Incidentally, as you would expect, walking over hilly terrain also burns more calories than walking on level ground. On the two days you don't walk, try to get in 20 minutes of strengthening exercises (see page 53).

Because you will undoubtedly do most of your walking outside, you have to be aware of the weather forecast and have a backup plan for inclement weather. On bad-weather days, you could use an indoor walking site (like a mall, or an indoor track), walk on a treadmill, or do stretching or strength exercises instead of walking.

Aerobic Exercise: A Jogging Program

If you are in reasonably good condition, have completed the "Walking Program for Beginners," or have been walking regularly, and have medical clearance, you can start a jogging program. Table 4.5 (on the following page) illustrates a 13-week beginner's schedule. Try to get your pulse into your TTZ but don't overdue it. Gradually, over time, you want to increase both the intensity and distance of your jogging routine. However, if you don't have the physical makeup to do both, always choose endurance over intensity; i.e., choose distance rather than speed, choose to jog longer rather than faster.

The first session in week 1 starts with approximately five minutes of walking at an easy pace of about 4 km/hr. Continue your warm up with two minutes of stretching. (See the stretching exercises outlined on pages 47 and 48.) Then start walking more briskly, about 6 km/hr, but check your pulse and increase or decrease this to get your heart rate close to a TTZ that is roughly consistent with a 45 percent intensity level. After five minutes of brisk walking, jog for three minutes at a slightly higher heart rate, corresponding to about a 55 percent intensity level. Continue with another five minutes of brisk walking and a three-minute jog. Cool down by walking again but now at an easy speed of about 4 km/hr for three minutes. Conclude your session by doing about two minutes of stretching. The total workout time in week 1 is 26 minutes per session. In weeks 2 through 13, the time allotted to brisk walking decreases as the jogging time gradually increases.

Jog at least three days a week for 13 weeks. Again, if you find a week particularly tiring, backup to the previous week (or repeat the week) before continuing with the program. Once you complete the program, if you want to improve, first go from jogging three days per week to five days per week – at the same TTZ. To improve further gradually increase your total workout time from 30 to 60 minutes. To improve even more, gradually increase your jogging speed, and TTZ, so that your exercise intensity level approaches 65 percent. Another good way to increase the intensity of your jogging workout is to try to include some hills in your workout. On the two days you don't walk, try to get in 20 minutes of strengthening exercises (See page 53.)

Week	Warm up (Minutes)		Brisk Walking & Jogging (Minutes)	Cool down (Minutes)		Total Minutes per Session
	Walk	Stretch		Walk	Stretch	
1	5	2	Walk 5 min, Jog 3 min Walk 5 min, Jog 3 min	3	2	26
2	5	2	Walk 4 min, Jog 5 min Walk 4 min, Jog 5 min	3	2	28
3	5	2	Walk 4 min, Jog 5 min Walk 4 min, Jog 5 min	3	2	28
4	5	2	Walk 4 min, Jog 6 min Walk 4 min, Jog 6 min	3	2	30
5	5	2	Walk 4 min, Jog 7min Walk 4 min, Jog 7 min	3	2	32
6	5	2	Walk 4 min, Jog 8 min Walk 4 min, Jog 8 min	3	2	34
7	5	2	Walk 4 min, Jog 9 min Walk 4 min, Jog 9 min	3	2	36
8	5	2	Walk 4 min, Jog 13 min Walk 4 min, Jog 13 min	3	2	27
9	5	2	Walk 4 min, Jog 15 min	3	2	29
10	5	2	Walk 4 min, Jog 17 min	3	2	31
11	5	2	Walk 2 min, Slow Jog 2 min then Jog 17 min	3	2	33
12	5	2	Walk 2 min, Slow Jog 3 min then Jog 17 min	3	2	34
13	5	2	Slow Jog 5 min then Jog 17 min	3	2	34

Table 4.5: Jogging Program for Beginners

Because you will undoubtedly do most of your jogging outside, you have to be aware of the weather forecast and have a contingency plan for inclement weather. On bad-weather days, you might use an indoor track, try an alternate exercise like jogging on a treadmill, or do stretching or strength exercises.

As always, stop exercising immediately if you experience tightness or pain in your chest, become lightheaded or dizzy, are severely breathless, lose muscle control or are nauseous. These are warning signs of over-exertion and you definitely should lower your exercise-intensity level. If you experience these symptoms, it is also a good idea to seek medical attention.

Be aware that the pounding your body gets from jogging usually takes its toll over time. Many joggers have recurring, nagging injuries, particularly to their legs and feet. If you begin to suffer chronic injuries, remember there are other high-intensity aerobic exercises for which your body might be better suited. At that point, you might consider switching to cycling, a rowing machine, etc. Before abandoning jogging altogether, however, you might want to cut back, and only jog two days per week and try another high-intensity, non-impact exercise the other three days of the week. Variety will also make your workout more enjoyable.

Your Body's Muscles

Your body has approximately 650 muscles that account for more than half your body weight. (You also have about 206 bones.) Figures 4.3 and 4.4, on the following pages, show the location of 17 of the muscles you will most likely hear trainers and health club members talking about as you workout. (Rather than pectorals, abdominals, deltoids, trapezius, latissimus dorsi, triceps, and biceps, you will probably hear more commonly used abbreviated versions, i.e., pecs, abs, delts, traps, lats, etcetera.) Many of these muscles are also referred to in the "Strength Programs" section that follows immediately. If you want to know more about your musculature, pick up a Human Anatomy and Physiology text at your local library.

Strength-Building Programs

As good as aerobic exercises are, they contribute little to building upper-body strength. And strength training can increase your muscle mass, which tends to increase your basal metabolic rate – and helps you control your weight.

If you are a beginner interested in strength training it's probably worthwhile to start by joining a health club, where you can get professional instruction on the proper use of exercise equipment, from dumbbells to rowing machines,

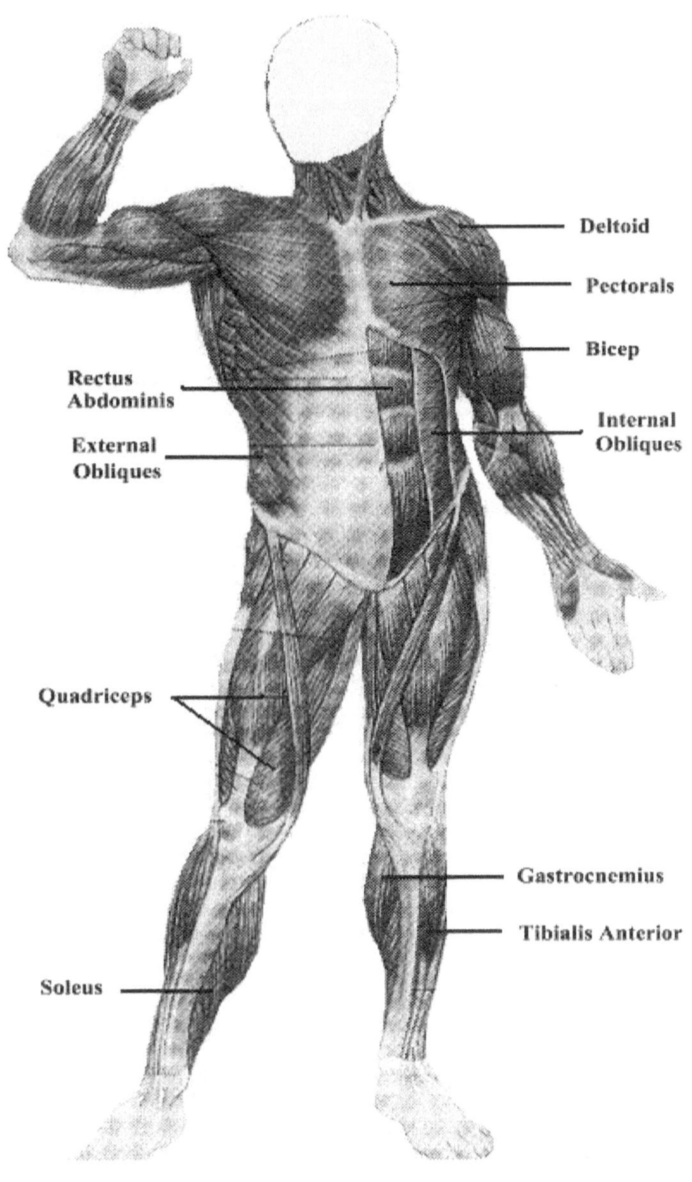

Figure 4.2: Human Body's Muscles – Front View

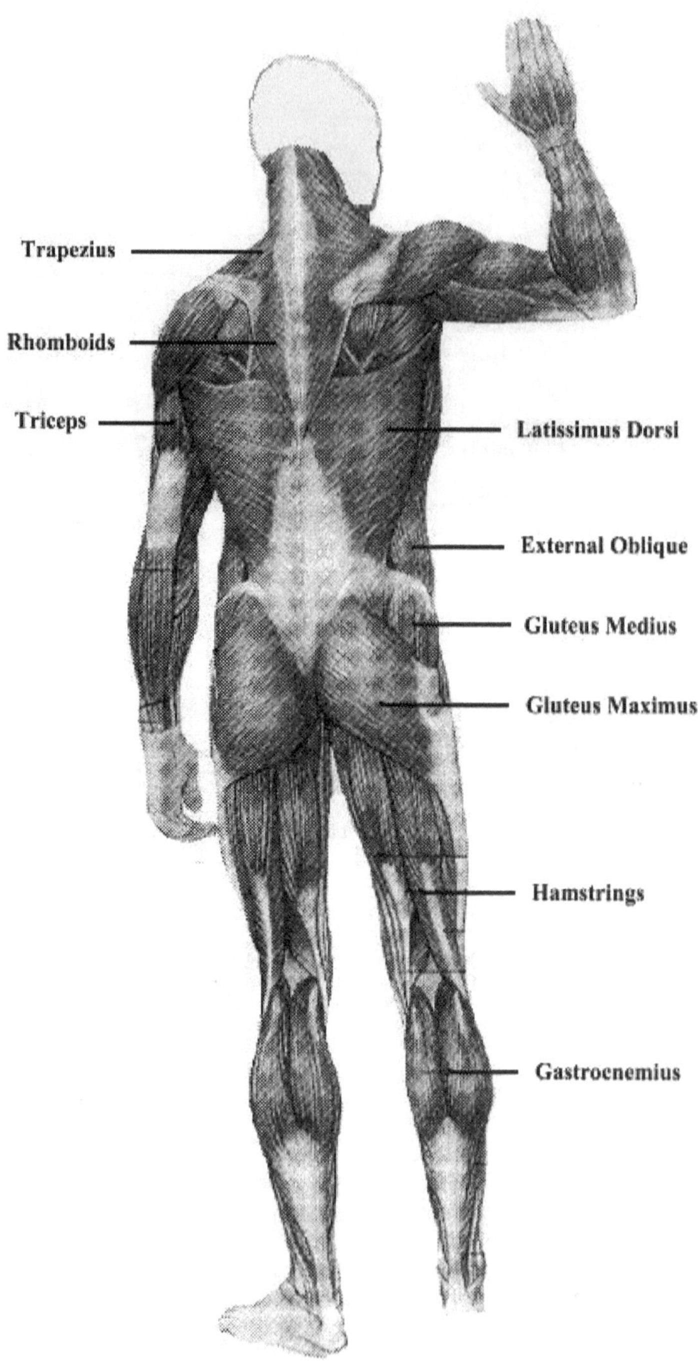

Figure 4.3: Human Body's Muscles – Rear View

and where you can compare different exercise routines. Another possibility is to hire a personal trainer for a couple of sessions to get you started on a program personalized to your fitness level and to teach you correct exercise techniques.

Of all the many strength-building options, I personally prefer free weights (actually dumbbells) because they can be used at home. Working out at home has some significant advantages. First, your workout takes less time because you don't have to drive back and forth to a fitness facility; second, you have the flexibility of dividing your workout into small time segments to fit your day, whenever you have time, such as when the baby is napping, and of course working out at home is certainly less expensive.

You can workout in a bedroom, basement, garage, attic – anywhere you have extra space. A set of variable (adjustable) weight dumbbells and a small weight bench don't take up much room and are all you need for a home-based gym. (Bear in mind, **knowledge and the discipline to work out regularly are far more important than fancy equipment**.) Before investing in a set of weights and a bench, however, it may still be worthwhile to start by joining a health club. At a health club you can get expert instruction on the use of free weights. And you may find that you actually prefer to workout at a club.

But if you do decide to opt for the convenience of a home-based gym, that would be the time to purchase a pair of variable-weight dumbbells and a strong weight bench (that will not tip over) for home use. Rather than an entire set of weights, purchase just enough dumbbell weight so that you can do a military press five times.

The seven dumbbell exercises that follow comprise a total-body workout, suitable for beginners, that involve all the major muscle groups. When done consecutively without stopping a series of exercises is called a circuit. To start, use the same dumbbell weight for all the exercises, a weight that allows you to do 10 to 15 repetitions of the most difficult exercise in the circuit. For the first week do one circuit per training session.

Your goal should be two circuits per session, which should take you about 20 minutes (with a two to three-minute rest between circuits). When you are comfortable at this level you are ready to increase the dumbbell weight – but by no more than roughly 10 percent (or one pound minimum). The seven exercises are illustrated in Figures 4.4 and 4.5. Perform 10 to 15 repetitions of each exercise.

a) <u>Bench Press</u>: With your head and back on the bench, hold a dumbbell in each hand to the side of your shoulders, palms facing each other. Slowly raise the dumbbells extending your arms above your shoulders. Pause, then lower the dumbbells down to the starting position. The bench press primarily works your pectorals, triceps and deltoids.

b) <u>One–Arm Dumbbell Row</u>: Hold a dumbbell in your right hand, palm facing toward your right thigh. Stand to the right of your weight bench and place your left knee on the bench. Support yourself by putting your left hand on the bench. (Flex your right knee slightly and lean forward so your back is almost parallel to the floor.) Slowly pull your right arm up until your upper arm is parallel to the floor. (Keep your right arm close to your torso.) Pause and lower your right arm to the starting position. After you complete a set, stand to the left of the bench and repeat the exercise with the dumbbell in your left hand. Rows mainly work your latissimus dorsi and rhomboid muscles.

c) <u>Seated Shoulder Press</u>: From a seated position, hold a dumbbell in each hand to the side of your shoulders, palms facing forward. Slowly raise the weights over your head until your arms are straight. Pause, then lower the dumbbells to the starting position. The shoulder press mainly exercises your deltoids, trapezius, triceps, latissimus dorsi and rhomboid muscles.

c) <u>Curls for Biceps</u>: Stand with a dumbbell in each hand, your arms hanging loosely, with your palms to the side your thighs and facing straight ahead. Keep your elbows tucked into your side and slowly lift the dumbbells until they are approximately shoulder high. Pause and lower the dumbbells to the starting position. Curls chiefly work your biceps.

e) <u>Tricep Extension</u>: With a dumbbell in your right hand, assume the same initial position as in the one-arm dumbbell row. Slowly move your right arm rearward until it is nearly parallel to the floor. Pause and then return the dumbbell to the starting position without bending your arm. After completing a set, stand to the left of the bench and repeat the exercise with the dumbbell in your left hand. This exercise mainly works your triceps.

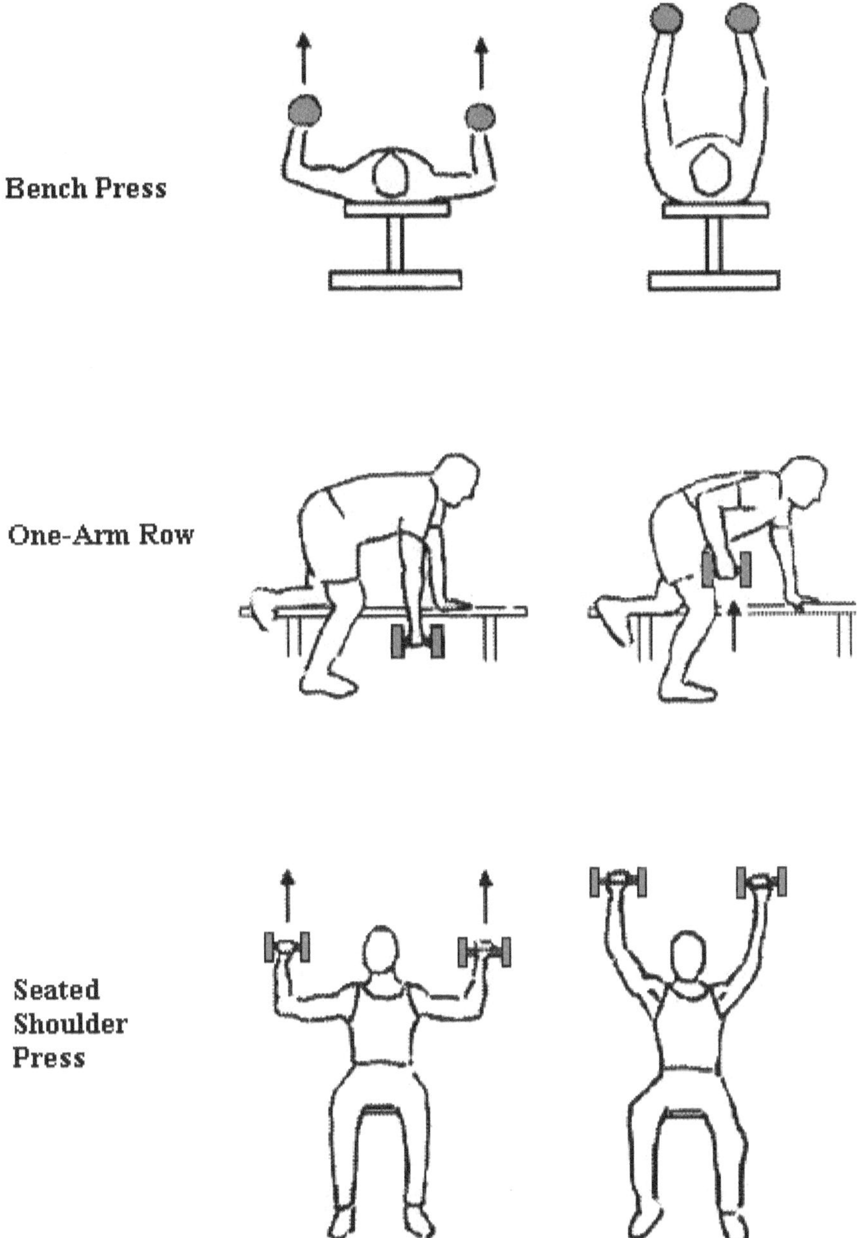

Figure 4.4: Strengthening Exercises (a to c)

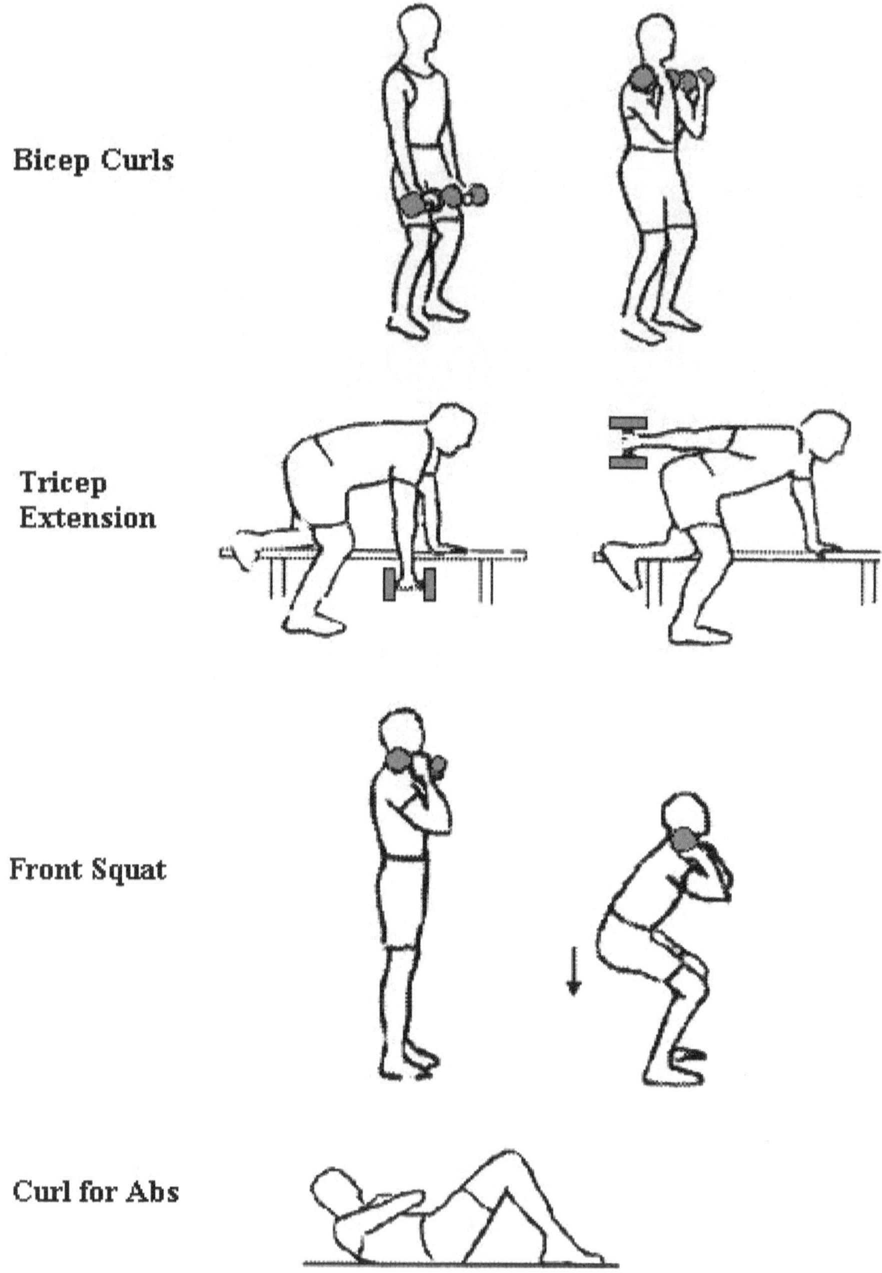

Figure 4.5: Strengthening Exercises (d to g)

f) <u>Front Squats</u>: Stand with a dumbbell in each hand, to the side of your shoulders, palms facing each other (inward). Slowly bend your knees and lower your body until your thighs are almost parallel to the floor. Try to keep your heels on the floor. Pause and gradually raise your body by straightening your knees. Squats work your gluteus, quadriceps and hamstrings.

g) <u>Curls for Abs</u>: This is not a weight lifting exercise but is a useful part of any routine. Lie face up on a floor mat with your hands folded over your chest and your legs bent. Keeping your feet flat on the mat, slowly curl your torso up and toward your thighs until your shoulder blades are off the mat. Pause, then return to the starting position. This exercise works your rectus abdominis muscles – your abs.

Remember to do about five minutes of aerobic and stretching exercises before and after your strength exercises, and to workout two to three (non-consecutive) days per week. Why non-consecutive days? Because strengthening exercises work a muscle until it's fatigued, and a day off is needed for muscles to recover, repair and rebuild. And remember to listen to your body to determine your level of exertion. Don't over do it!

A final word about breathing properly: Never hold your breath during weight training. This can cause your blood pressure to get dangerously high. Rather, breathe naturally and try to exhale during a lift.

Additional Strength-Building Exercises

As your conditioning improves, you may want a more challenging workout. This can be accomplished in a number of ways. One method is to use two pairs of variable weight dumbbells, with a different weight loaded on each set of dumbbells. Now, you can more closely equalize the difficulty of the different exercises by using the lighter pair for harder exercises and the heavier pair of dumbbells for easier exercises. Yet another way to make your workout more demanding is to add one or more of the following exercises to your routine:

h) <u>Dumbbell Fly (not illustrated)</u>: With your head and back on the bench, hold a dumbbell in each hand and fully extend your arms upward with your palms facing each other. Keeping your arms fully extended, slowly lower the dumbbells sideways to chest level. Pause, then return the dumbbells to the starting position. The dumbbell fly primarily trains your pectorals, triceps and deltoids.

i) <u>Dumbbell Pullover (not illustrated)</u>: With your head and back on the bench, hold a dumbbell in each hand and fully extend your arms upward with your palms facing each other. Allow your arms to bend as you lower the dumbbells behind your head. Pause, then return the dumbbells to the starting position. The dumbbell pullover primarily works your triceps and deltoids.

j) <u>Standing Back Press (not illustrated)</u>: Stand with your feet about 12 inches apart. Hold a dumbbell in each hand at shoulder height and slightly behind your shoulders, with your palms facing forward. Slowly raise the weights over your head until your arms are straight. Pause, then lower the dumbbells to the starting position. The shoulder press mainly works your deltoids, trapezius, triceps, latissimus dorsi and rhomboid muscles.

k) <u>Knee-Bend Kicks (not illustrated)</u>: Sit on the floor and lean back supporting some of your weight on your forearms. Raise both heals about three inches off the floor. Flex and lift your right leg. Return your right leg to its starting position. Then do the flex and lift with your left leg. Repeat as often as you can. This floor exercise works your abdominals.

Other Exercises

There are literally hundreds of other aerobic, flexibility and strengthening exercises. Too many to review here, but many are definitely worth considering. For instance, swimming laps in a pool provides an excellent low-impact aerobic workout that also builds strength. Of course, the disadvantage is that you need to join a fitness facility that has a pool. Some trainers think a good rowing machine, such as the Concept II, provides a great total-body workout. Others feel a workout on a stairclimber is hard to beat. All have advantages and disadvantages.

In fact, most trainers recommend that you modify your routine every few months to add variety. Some advocate alternating exercises every other session. For instance, if you jog and lift weights on alternate days, you avoid repeating movements on consecutive days. As bonus, you will also most likely avoid the injuries that are often associated with day-after-day repetitive motion.

What if You Miss a Workout?

Inevitably, you will miss some workouts. It may be due to a heavy work schedule, a minor illness, or an injury. If you are injured or ill, wait for the injury to heal, or for when you feel like your normal self before resuming your exercise routine.

If you only miss a day or two, you can undoubtedly just pick up where you left off as if nothing happened. If you miss a week or more, however, you will probably have lost some of your fitness gains and might have to resume at a somewhat lower exercising-intensity level. This means that when you come back after missing some aerobic sessions, you might have to exercise at a slightly lower TTZ, or shorten the duration of your workout. And when you return after missing some strengthening sessions, you might want to reduce the weight you are lifting or reduce the number of repetitions.

Incidentally, physical fitness can be maintained only by regular workouts. If your exercise frequency drops to one day a week, half your fitness gains will be lost in 10 weeks. If exercise is stopped completely, virtually all your accumulated fitness benefits will be lost in five weeks! Therefore, if you want to keep that state of well-being, feeling better, looking better, it's important to make regular aerobic exercise part of your lifestyle.

Exercising in Hot Weather

When you engage in vigorous exercise, your body generates a great deal of heat, and your body temperature can rise from 37°C up to 38.5°C. (A body temperature of 40.5°C is life threatening.)

High ambient temperatures and high humidity are a concern because both influence how effectively you transfer the heat your body generates to the environment. High ambient temperatures are an obvious cooling problem, but high levels of humidity also cause cooling difficulties by hindering the evaporation of perspiration. As a result, on days when it is both hot and humid it is even more difficult to transfer heat from your body to the surrounding ambient air. This combination can cause your body temperature to rise to dangerous levels. **On hot humid summer days, therefore, you must guard against overdoing it**.

Heat Index: Adopted by the U.S. National Weather Service, the heat index, or apparent temperature, combines the effects of air (dry bulb) temperature and relative humidity. (Heat index values are expressed in either degrees Fahrenheit or Celsius.) The heat index is not perfect but it is the best available guide for the general population. As expected, Table 4.6 shows that when the heat index rises, so do health risks. In hot weather, the major health threats are heat stroke, heat exhaustion and dehydration.

Category	Heat Index		Heat-Related Risks
	(°F)	(°C)	
Caution	80 to 90°F	27 to 32°C	Unexpected fatigue possible with prolonged exposure and/or physical activity.
Extreme Caution	90 to 105°F	32 to 41°C	Muscle cramps and/or heat exhaustion possible with prolonged exposure and/or physical activity.
Danger	105 to 129°F	41 to 54°C	Muscle cramps and/or heat exhaustion likely. Heat stroke possible with long exposure and/or physical activity.
Extreme Danger	130°F or higher	54°C or higher	Heat stroke likely.

Table 4.6: Health Risks vs. Hot Weather Conditions (Heat Index)

Heat Exhaustion: As described in Table 4.6, when heat index values reach 32 to 41°C, you could suffer muscle cramps, particularly in your legs and heat exhaustion. The symptoms of heat exhaustion are pale clammy skin, dizziness or fainting, a rapid pulse, fast breathing, and nausea. If you experience any of these problems, get to a cool place, lie down and sip water. You may also need to seek medical attention.

Heat Stroke: Much more dangerous is heat stroke, which results when extremely hot weather triggers a malfunction of the body's thermostat, causing the body temperature to rise to 40°C or higher. Symptoms of heat stroke are confusion or loss of consciousness, flushed, hot and dry skin, a strong and rapid pulse. **Heat stroke is a medical emergency**. Move the person to the coolest accessible place and call 911. Some first aid measures include removing some of the person's clothing and sponging with cool water.

Dehydration: Everyone knows drinking water is important for good health, but it's even more important on hot days while you are exercising. During vigorous exercise, you can lose one to two quarts of water per hour in sweat, so it's essential to use common sense and stay hydrated. And in hot weather, drink plenty of water and fruit juice even if you don't feel thirsty.

Relative Humidity (%)	Air Temperature (°C)											
	28	30	32	34	36	38	40	42	44	46	48	50
10	27	28	30	32	33	35	37	39	41	43	45	48
15	27	28	30	32	34	36	38	41	43	46	49	52
20	27	28	30	32	34	37	39	42	46	49	53	57
25	27	28	30	33	35	38	41	45	48	53	57	62
30	27	29	31	33	36	39	43	47	52	57	62	
35	27	29	32	34	38	41	46	50	56	61		
40	28	30	32	35	39	43	48	54	60	66		
45	28	30	33	37	41	46	51	58	64			
50	28	31	34	38	43	49	55	62				
55	29	32	36	40	46	52	59	66				
60	30	33	37	42	48	55	63					
65	30	34	39	44	51	59	67					
70	31	35	40	47	54	63						
75	31	36	42	49	58	67						
80	32	38	44	52	61				Note: Exposure to full sun can increase heat index by 8°C.			
85	33	39	47	55	65							
90	34	41	49	58								
95	35	42	52	62								
100	36	44	54									

Table 4.7: Heat Index for Various Temperature-Humidity Combinations Duns

Another annoying problem in hot weather is chafing. Skin irritation can happen anywhere clothing touches your skin. If you are bothered by this troubling condition try different clothing styles, fabrics, or simply coat the affected area with petroleum jelly.

Before exercising outdoors in hot weather, check your latest local weather forecast. If the forecast does not incorporate the heat index, you can use the forecasted air temperature and relative humidity to determine a heat index value using Table 4.7. (Note the heat index values in Table 4.7 are in degrees Celsius and the colours in the table correspond to those in the risk categories shown in Table 4.6.)

Frankly, unless you are relatively young and in very good physical condition, **it is not a good idea to engage in vigorous outdoor exercise when the heat index is over 33°C**. Despite this advice, if you persist on exercising on very hot days, make sure you wear loose-fitting, light-collared clothes; avoid the blazing sun (which can increase the heat index by 8°C) by working out early in the morning or the evening; wear a hat and use sun screen; reduce the intensity of your workout; and drink plenty of water. In addition, be aware that the temperature of paved roadways can easily exceed 38°C even when the ambient air temperature is only 26°C. Therefore, if you are intent on jogging on hot days it is best to do so in a shaded park. Finally when you workout in very hot weather always let someone know when and where you will be exercising and what time you plan to return.

Exercising in Cold Weather

The ideal exercise temperature range is about 4 to 29°C with a wind speed less than 25 kph, but many people continue to exercise outdoors at temperatures well below 4°C. Generally, cold weather is less dangerous to an exerciser – but definitely not risk-free. When you exercise outdoors in cold weather you encounter an entirely new set of difficulties. Besides often-treacherous footing on snow-covered or icy surfaces, you must contend with low temperatures and the wind.

Wind Chill Temperature Index: Basic physics states that when heat leaves an object the temperature of the object drops. The same principle applies to your body. As heat leaves your body, your temperature drops and you feel cold. Very low ambient temperatures combined with the wind increase the amount of heat leaving your body. As the wind speed increases, the temperature of any exposed skin drops even further. The Wind Chill Temperature Index was developed in an effort to quantify this phenomenon,

and is a measure of the relative discomfort due to combined cold temperature and wind. In essence, the wind-chill temperature lets you know what the outside air temperature "feels like," based on the heat loss from skin exposed to low air temperatures and the wind.

In 2010, the U.S. National Weather Service and Environment Canada jointly issued a new Wind Chill Temperature Index. Table 4.8 presents a version of the Wind Chill Temperature Index issued by the U.S. National Weather Service. (The wind-chill temperatures in Table 4.8 are in degrees Celsius and the colours in the table correspond to those in the risk categories shown in Table 4.9. Note that exposure to bright sunshine helps, because the sun may increase wind-chill temperatures by 5 to 10°C. The combination of low air temperatures and increasing wind speeds can result in incredibly low wind-chill temperatures. For instance, Table 4.8 shows that an air temperature of -34°C and a wind speed of 60 kph produces a wind chill temperature of -56°C. Now that's cold! And dangerous!

One of the **potential consequences of very low wind chill temperatures is frostbite**. Table 4.9 (on page 69) employs the Canadian interpretation of frostbite risks rather than the U.S. version. (After all, who knows more about cold weather than Canadians?) **Other serious cold weather related conditions are hypothermia and heart attack.**

Frostbite: When body tissue freezes the injury is called frostbite, which usually strikes fingers, toes, nose and ears. Frostbitten skin is numb, hard and pale, and requires immediate medical attention. If you suspect you have frostbite, get indoors as quickly as you can and call or send for help. First aid steps include covering the frozen area with a blanket and drinking a warm non-alcoholic beverage.

Hypothermia: Prolonged exposure to extreme cold, especially during exercise, can result in a depletion of energy stores (calories) which can cause a drop in body temperature. This in turn can cause a gradual mental slowing. The stricken person becomes increasingly unreasonable, clumsy, irritable, sleepy, and eventually lapses into a coma. This is a life-threatening condition. (Severe hypothermia can lead to cardiac and respiratory failure and death.) To help, your first move should be to call your local emergency phone number for help. Then start first aid (which is beyond the scope of this book).

Heart Attack: As the air temperature drops, your body's air-warming system may not be able to adequately heat the cold air entering your mouth and flowing down your windpipe. As a result, the incoming cold air may cause your coronary arteries to constrict – resulting in a heart attack – particularly if you are not in good condition.

Air Temp (°C)	Wind Speed (kph)										
	0	10	20	30	40	50	60	70	80	90	100
4	4	2	0	-1	-2	-3	-3	-4	-4	-5	-5
2	2	-1	-3	-4	-5	-5	-6	-7	-7	-7	-8
0	0	-3	-5	-7	-7	-8	-9	-9	-10	-10	-11
-2	-2	-6	-8	-9	-10	-11	-12	-12	-13	-13	-14
-4	-4	-8	-10	-12	-13	-14	-14	-15	-16	-16	-16
-6	-6	-11	-13	-14	-15	-16	-17	-18	-18	-19	-19
-8	-8	-13	-15	-17	-18	-19	-20	-21	-21	-22	-22
-10	-10	-15	-18	-20	-21	-22	-23	-23	-24	-25	-25
-12	-12	-18	-20	-22	-23	-25	-25	-26	-27	-27	-28
-14	-14	-20	-23	-25	-26	-27	-28	-29	-30	-30	-31
-16	-16	-22	-25	-27	-29	-30	-31	-32	-33	-33	-34
-18	-18	-25	-28	-30	-31	-33	-34	-35	-35	-36	-37
-20	-20	-27	-30	-33	-34	-35	-36	-37	-38	-39	-40
-22	-22	-30	-33	-35	-37	-38	-39	-40	-41	-42	-43
-24	-24	-32	-36	-38	-39	-41	-42	-43	-44	-45	-45
-26	-26	-34	-38	-40	-42	-44	-45	-46	-47	-48	-48
-28	-28	-37	-41	-43	-45	-46	-48	-49	-50	-50	-51
-30	-30	-39	-43	-46	-48	-49	-50	-51	-52	-53	-54
-32	-32	-42	-46	-48	-50	-52	-53	-54	-55	-56	-57
-34	-34	-44	-48	-51	-53	-54	-56	-57	-58	-59	-60
-36	-36	-46	-51	-53	-56	-57	-59	-60	-61	-62	-63
-38	-38	-49	-53	-56	-58	-60	-61	-63	-64	-65	-66
-40	-40	-51	-56	-59	-61	-63	-64	-65	-67	-68	-69

Table 4.8: Wind-Chill Temperature vs. Air Temperature & Wind Speed

One of the **potential consequences of very low wind-chill temperatures is frostbite**. Table 4.9 (on the next page) employs the Canadian interpretation of frostbite risks rather than the U.S. version. (After all, who knows more about cold weather than Canadians?) **Other serious cold weather related conditions are hypothermia and heart attack.**

Frostbite: When body tissue freezes the injury is called frostbite, which usually strikes fingers, toes, nose and ears. Frostbitten skin is numb, hard and pale, and requires immediate medical attention. If you suspect you have frostbite, get indoors as quickly as you can and call or send for help. First aid steps include covering the frozen area with a blanket and drinking a warm nonalcoholic beverage.

Wind Chill Temperature	Frostbite Risk for Most People	Exposure Time
4°C to -27°C	Low	---
-28°C to -37°C	Medium	10 to 30 minutes
-37°C to -47°C	High	5 to 10 minutes
-48°C to -53°C	Higher	2 to 5 minutes
-54°C to -67°C	Highest	2 minutes or less

Table 4.9: Frostbite Risk vs. Wind-Chill Temperature

Hypothermia: Prolonged exposure to extreme cold, especially during exercise, can result in a depletion of energy stores (calories) which can cause a drop in body temperature. This in turn can cause gradual mental slowing. The stricken person becomes increasingly unreasonable, clumsy, irritable, sleepy, and eventually lapses into a coma.   This is a life-threatening condition. Severe hypothermia can lead to cardiac and respiratory failure and death. To help, your first move should be to call 911.   Then start first aid (which is beyond the scope of this book).

Heart Attack: As the air temperature drops, your body's air-warming system may not be able to adequately heat the cold air entering your mouth and flowing down your windpipe. As a result, the incoming cold air may cause your coronary arteries to constrict – resulting in a heart attack – particularly if you are not in good condition.

Upshot of Cold Weather: Once the wind-chill temperature reaches approximately 10°F exercising outdoors becomes increasingly uncomfortable. Even if you are an outdoor enthusiast, at this wind chill you may want to think about changing to an indoor exercise routine until the weather moderates.

At a wind chill temperature of approximately -28°C the risk of frostbite starts to increase. Unless you are skiing cross-country or downhill, or engaged in another winter sport that requires you to be outdoors, in bitterly-cold weather, the best advice is to exercise indoors. Furthermore, it is **not a good idea to exercise outdoors when the wind-chill temperature is below -30°C**. At this wind chill temperature any exposed skin will freeze in about 20 minutes. In brief then, even if you are relatively young and in very good condition, rather than exercising outdoors in very cold weather, consider joining a health club, setting up a small workout space at your home, or walking in an enclosed mall.

Upshot of Cold Weather: Once the wind-chill temperature reaches approximately -12°C exercising outdoors becomes increasingly uncomfortable. Even if you are an outdoor enthusiast, at this wind chill you may want to think about changing to an indoor exercise routine until the weather moderates.

Dressing for Cold Weather: Notwithstanding our best advice, if you still intend to exercise outdoors in frigid weather, wear layers of loose-fitting, lightweight, warm clothing. The layer closest to your skin should be a thin layer of a synthetic wicking material that draws perspiration away from your body. The second layer should provide insulation. Water-resistant fleece is a good option. Your third, outer layer, should be windproof and waterproof with a hood. Generally, mittens are warmer than gloves, and wool or polypropylene socks insulate and wick moisture. Wear a head sock that covers your entire head and neck with openings only for breathing and vision. Consider covering your mouth with a scarf to cause the air you breathe to be slightly warmer and more humid. Further, wear goggles or wraparound sunglasses to protect your eyes from wind and ultraviolet radiation. And make sure to stay dry.

In addition, remember to drink plenty of water – even in cold weather – to make up for water you lose when you sweat during vigorous exercise.

Exercise Risks and Problems

Certain situations may occur that indicate you may be doing too much, exercising too hard. For example, regardless of your pulse rate you should never be left completely breathless by your aerobic exercise. A good rule to remember is: **You are exercising too hard if you cannot carry on a conversation while you are jogging, cycling, etcetera**. A feeling of having worked hard is fine, sweating is good, but not a feeling of undo fatigue.

Perhaps the most frequent problems faced by exercisers are injuries of the joints and muscles: sprains and strains, knee pain, elbow pain, back pain, neck pain, shin splints and stress fractures. Most happen when you exercise too hard.

Potentially serious problems are signaled if you experience any of the following symptoms during or after exercise. The symptoms include but are not limited to any abnormal heart action such as an irregular heart rhythm; pain or pressure in the middle of your chest; pain in an arm or your neck; dizziness, fainting or lightheadedness; severe exhaustion; sudden loss of coordination; or confusion. If any of these symptoms are experienced, stop exercising immediately and get medical help.

How to Avoid Injury

Before he retired, my long-time friend and mentor, Dr. Kanaar's specialty was rehabilitation medicine but he also preached what he called "preventive medicine," that is avoiding injury by practicing a common-sense approach to exercise:

- **Have a medical checkup and then set realistic fitness goals.**

- **Build up your exercise intensity gradually over many weeks, months.**

- **After you eat a meal, wait two hours before exercising.**

- **Buy good suitable for your exercise routine.**

- **Use safety and protective equipment when appropriate, such as helmet when you bicycle, and goggles when you play handball, squash or racquetball.**

- **On hot days, follow the precautions in the section "Exercising in Hot Weather."**

- **On cold days, follow the precautions in the section "Exercising in Cold Weather."**

- **If you insist on working out in very hot or cold weather, always let someone know when and where you will be exercising and when you are planning to return.**

- **If you are new to a gym or health club, attend an orientation session before you use any unfamiliar exercise equipment. Otherwise, read the operating instructions carefully and ask someone qualified to help you.**

- **For aerobic activities, warm up slowly to reach your TTZ and cool down slowly after you exercise.**

- **Do not increase the difficulty of any activity (e.g., your walking or jogging distance, the amount of weight you lift) by more than 10 percent per week.**

- **Jog on softer surfaces such as a level grass field, a dirt path, or a running track.**

- **After exercising wait 30 minutes before eating.**

- **As a final point, if you experience some early warning pain stop exercising.**

Many minor leg injuries of the muscles and joints can be easily treated using the well-known R.I.C.E. method, i.e., rest, ice, compression, elevation.

Rest. You may not have to avoid all physical activity; just taking it easy might be fine.

Ice. Apply ice for 15 minutes several times a day for as long as there is any swelling.

Compress the area with a bandage or sleeve to help control swelling.

Elevate the injured area above the level of your heart.

On the other hand, if early pain is ignored and you continue exercising, a minor injury may become more serious.

Keep an Exercise Log

Individuals who keep a record of their exercise generally exercise more often and have more success over the long term. How should you go about this? Keep an exercise log. A sample Daily Exercise Log is shown in Table 4.10 (on the next page) with two days filled in.

Day	Aerobic Exercise	Distance	Time	Heart Rate	Strength Exercise	Weight	Reps	Sets
Mon 11/06 /	Walking	6.5 km	65 min	124	None			
Tues 11/07	Walking	6.75 km	72 min	122	Bench Press	5 kg	12	2
					Rows	8 kg	12	2
					Tricep Extension	5 kg	12	2
					Press	8 kg	12	2
					Curls	8 kg	12	2
					Squats	8 kg	10	1
					Abs	N/A	25	2

Table 4.10: Sample Exercise Log

One Fitness Expert's Ideal Exercise

A prominent 43-year-old professor of physiology was asked at the end of a speech to a group of business executives to give her definition of the "ideal" exercise. Without hesitation she reeled off her checklist, saying her ideal exercise would be one which:

- Is aerobic, preferably where the arms as well as the legs are used.

- Is efficient, yielding the maximum fitness return for the minimum time investment.

- Can be done every day if desired, outside or indoors, i.e., is not weather dependent.

- Does not require any special equipment or facilities.

- Requires only one participant.

- Is fun!

She went on to tell of her extremely busy schedule: laboratory research, classroom teaching, speaking engagements, consulting. Yet she said she exercised every day virtually without fail, whether teaching in Chicago, visiting her publisher in New York City, or speaking in St. Louis. She bragged that her total time expenditure on overt exercise was usually only 40 minutes a day.

Then she described the exercise program she now follows that she felt most closely met her ideal. She said she was a "morning person" and that she got in her daily exercise first thing in the morning. She warmed up by doing stretching exercises for a few minutes, and then while watching the morning news on television she jogged in place for 30 minutes – making sure her pulse reached approximately 145 beats per minute - high enough to put her at the 70% exercise intensity level. She did a few sets of push-ups, abdominal curls and finally more stretching as she cooled off. Then still perspiring she jumped into the shower, she would have taken anyway, toweled off and was ready for breakfast. She added that when she was home she also jogged in place, and for variety every other day she rode a stationary bike. She exercised every day.

In conclusion, she admitted that her real passion was tennis which she played whenever she could, but which she said was only an adjunct to her exercise program not the backbone. Her reason: She could not reasonably expect to fit at least three or four tennis workouts a week into her schedule. Arranging for courts and partners, driving to the tennis courts, changing clothes, taking a needed extra shower, the entire process took more than two hours per session. Besides, a good deal of the time she missed her tennis match because she was out of town or too busy to take the time!

My Exercise Routine

I started jogging in the late 1960's. Of course I was much younger then. I jogged five to eight kilometres almost every morning and worked out with free weights (dumbbells) on the days I didn't jog. After 20 years of jogging, the constant pounding resulted in a troubling number of chronic minor leg and foot injuries. So I switched to walking and I have been walking ever since. Now I'm a semi-retired senior citizen; so I have more time than most. For the past 15 years, from 6:00 to 7:00 am, I take a brisk walk covering 6.5 kilometres. Most days I walk outside but when the weather is bad I head for a nearby shopping mall. For variety, every other day, I power walk in place for about 45 minutes using one of my six exercise DVDs to set the rhythm; then I complete my workout doing two circuits of the dumbbell exercises described starting on page 54.

In warmer weather I golf (walk 9 or 18 holes) or hike (about eight miles) two or three times a week. On those days – that's my workout. Although just a week before this writing, I finished my brisk one-hour morning walk followed by 20 minutes of dumbbell exercises. Then later in the day a friend called and next thing I know I'm playing 18 holes of golf. Walking – of course. In total, I exercised 5 hours and 45 minutes, burned about 2000 Calories, and felt strong, definitely not tired, at the end of the day. Not bad for a senior!

In summary, one day I walk outside for an hour; the following day I power walk in place for 40 minutes using an exercise DVD and also lift weights; the next day I'm back to walking outside again; and so on. I've been doing this for 15 years. I exercise every day without fail. Every day!
And because walking is the central part of my program, I almost never suffer an exercise-related injury.

My exercise routine combined with a sensible diet have kept me trim over the years (within three pounds of my college-graduation weight). Most people think I'm much younger than my chronological age – and I feel great!

Workout to Feel Good & Get Healthy
If your goal is a chiseled body with washboard abs and the endurance and strength of a triathlon athlete, you're reading the wrong book. Sure the aerobic and strength routines outlined here will help you get in shape, slim down and get somewhat stronger – but your body is not going to be transformed into the physique of a world-class athlete.

This chapter is about how you should workout to get fit so that you feel good and stay healthy. And you're not going to get fit just because you join a fancy health club with lots of high-tech equipment – if you only workout

 once or twice a week, or every other week. Joining a health club is great – if you use it consistently.

The words that describe our kind of workout are consistent, determined, steady, persistent, dogged, unswerving, gritty, single-minded. Get the point? In our kind of workout, you decide that you will workout at least five days a week; that an aerobic exercise will form the core of your workout, and that you will incorporate some strengthening exercises two days a week. After that, it doesn't matter exactly what exercises you choose, what equipment you use, or what facility you use. These are secondary factors. What matters most is that you exercise consistently. **To improve muscle tone and overall fitness, feel good and stay healthy, you should exercise at least five days per week, day after day, week after week, year after year – for as long as you are physically able.** Remember the key words: consistent, determined, steady, persistent, dogged, unswerving, gritty, single-minded. Consistent!

5. LIFE-LONG FITNESS

There are lots of reasons to get fit: a longer life expectancy, less illness, a healthful appearance, the ability to work (and play) with vigor and an energy reserve for emergencies. To repeat what was said earlier, people who undertake a physical fitness program and attain a heightened level of fitness, report a dramatic reduction in chronic fatigue, an improved ability to relax, more energy for day-to-day tasks, firmer muscles and increased strength. In short, they feel better and look better too!

Why then is it so easy to become a dropout when fitness offers such wonderful health benefits? A good plan may be the missing link to getting and staying fit. My friend and mentor Dr. Kanaar was a wonderful swimmer. Many years ago, he not only taught me to be a more efficient swimmer, but at the same time he convinced me that it was especially **important for an individual starting a physical fitness program to set goals, have a plan and keep a fitness log.**

Set Goals, Have a Plan & Keep a Log

Everyone's personal goals and plan of attack will be different. Let us assume your goals are to lose 20 pounds and improve your overall health and fitness. First, commit yourself and start immediately. (Buy a notebook, or use your computer, because you will need to put your goals and plans in writing.) Next, plan how you are going to attain these goals. Broadly speaking, your overall plan might be to stop smoking; to begin a weight loss diet; and to start exercising. You must, however, be more specific and develop a detailed plan that indicates the when and how you are going to stop smoking, lose weight, etcetera. You might make up your mind to stop "cold turkey," or to enter a smoking secession program. Note the date you plan to start and the date you expect to be smoke free. Put it in writing!

For the weight loss portion of your plan, decide if you are going to go it alone or join some sort of clinical or non-clinical program. [Incidentally, all the information you need for a do-it-yourself weight loss program can be found in *Weight Control - U.S. Edition* published by NoPaperPress.] If you settle on a do-it-yourself program, again note the diet calorie level, milestone dates for weight loss, etcetera. Put it in writing!

Then choose an exercise routine. Again using the principles covered in this book devise a realistic plan with time, place, type of exercise and frequency. Put it writing!

By now you must appreciate why you need a notebook. Once you actually start implementing your plan, you should also keep an exercise log and a food log to record your progress. An all-in-one fitness log that includes exercise as well as food is illustrated in Table 5.1 on the next page. As you progress, periodically update your fitness plan. Enlist the support of your family and friends and do not forget to reward yourself when you reach a milestone – for a job well done!

The Keys to Life-Long Fitness

As with most pursuits, the earlier in life you begin the better. But regardless of your age, the sooner you start a fitness program the easier it will be to get in shape and the more time you will have to reap the benefits. So for less illness, for a longer life expectancy, for a healthful appearance, start on the path to physical fitness now!

Despite all the detailed information presented in this book the path to life-long fitness is actually deceptively simple, and can be reduced to five basic keys. Assuming you have had a medical checkup, the five basic keys to life-long fitness are:

Key 1: Stop smoking and limit the consumption of alcoholic beverages. For some this will be difficult but both are absolutely necessary for life-long fitness.

Key 2: Keep your weight under control. Know your maintenance calorie value, i.e., how many calories you can eat to neither gain nor lose weight. Periodically you might experience a noteworthy weight gain. If this happens go on a mini-diet. [See *Total Weight Control - U.S. Edition*.]

Key 3: Practice good nutrition by eating a variety of foods from each food group – all within your caloric allowance. [Again, see *Total Weight Control - U.S. Edition*.]

Key 4: Engage in some form of moderate strength training at least two non-consecutive days per week.

Key 5: Engage in some form of moderate aerobic exercise every single day of the year. That is right every day! (If need be, cut back your aerobic workout on the days you do your strength exercises.)

Meal	Foods	Amount	kcalories	Comments
Breakfast	Juice Cereal Skim milk Black coffee	125 mL 30 g 125 mL	55 110 40	Orange Juice Wheat cereal
Snack	Tea		0	
Mid-day Meal	Cottage cheese Broccoli Whole wheat bread	225 g 50 g 1 slice	160 25 75	Fat free
Snack	Cracker or biscuit Tea		60	
Evening Meal	Salmon Baked potato Green salad + olive oil Mixed veggies Apple Whole wheat bread Skim milk	125 g Medium 15 mL 50 g Medium 1 slice 250 mL	200 100 140 40 75 75 80	Total of 1235 kcal
Snack	Tea		0	

Strength Exercise	Dumbbell Weight	Reps	Sets	Aerobic Exercise	Distance	Time	Heart Rate
Bench Press	5 kg	12	2	Walking	6.75 km	72mi	124
Rows	7 kg	12	2				
Tricep Ext	5 kg	12	2				
Press	5 kg	12	2				
Curls	7 kg	12	2				
Squats	7 kg	10	1				
Abs	N/A	25	2				

Table 5.1: Sample All-In-One Fitness Log for Tuesday July 11th

Sure, there will be some days when it may seem impossible to fit exercise into your hectic schedule. Everyone would like to be able to workout for an uninterrupted hour, but the good news is that studies have shown that workouts as short as 15 minutes can improve your health. So on those very hectic, crazy days, try to fit in several 15-minute workouts whenever you can. Do the best with the time you have.

Any other occasional additional exercise such as a round of golf on the weekend, a game of handball, cross-country skiing, attending a yoga class, is fine, beneficial, but should be considered secondary to your daily aerobic workout.

Now It's Up To You

At this point, you have everything you need to succeed. You have an understanding of the fundamentals of exercise, nutrition and weight control. You have set realistic fitness goals, and you have a good fitness plan. If you combine all these with intense desire you'll be unstoppable. Your fitness regimen will work wonders and will have you looking and feeling better both physically and mentally. And when you look and feel your best, your spirit will soar.

So as you start on the road to fitness, be aware that you are well prepared for success and always keep in mind how good you'll feel when you reach your goals.

So what are you waiting for? Make it happen! Good luck!

<u>NoPaperPress Paperbacks and eBooks</u>

100-Day Super Diet-1200 Calorie*	Weight Loss for Men - Metric*
100-Day Super Diet-1500 Calorie*	Maximum Weight Loss- 1200 Calorie*
100-Day No-Cooking Diet-1200 Cal*	Maximum Weight Loss- 1500 Calorie*
100-Day No-Cooking Diet-1500 Cal*	Weight Control - U.S. Edition
90-Day Smart Diet-1200 Calorie*	Weight Control - Metric. Edition
90-Day Smart Diet-1500 Calorie*	Professional Weight Control Women - U.S.
90-Day No-Cooking Diet - 1200 Cal*	Professional Weight Control Women - Metric
90-Day No-Cooking Diet - 1500 Cal*	Professional Weight Control Men - U.S.
90-Day Perfect Diet - 1200 Calorie*	Professional Weight Control Men - Metric
90-Day Perfect Diet - 1500 Calorie*	Weight Maintenance - U.S. Edition*
60-Day Perfect Diet-1200 Calorie*	Weight Maintenance - Metric. Edition*
60-Day Perfect Diet-1500 Calorie*	Weight Maintenance - UK Edition
50-Day Flex Diet-1200 Calorie*	Weight Loss for Senior Men*
50-Day Flex Diet-1500 Calorie*	Weight Loss for Senior Women*
30-Day Quick Diet - for Women*	Eat Smart - U.S. Edition*
30-Day Quick Diet - for Men*	Eat Smart - Metric Edition
30-Day No-Cooking Diet*	30-Day Mediterranean Diet
30-Day Diet for Women - Metric*	Exercise Smart - U.S. Edition*
30-Day Diet for Men - Metric*	Exercise Smart - Metric Edition
25 Day Easy Diet-1200 Calorie*	Exercise Smart - UK Edition*
25 Day Easy Diet-1500 Calorie*	Total Fitness - U.S. Edition
25-Day No-Cooking Diet	Total Fitness - Metric Edition
10-Day Express Diet	Total Fitness - UK Edition
10-Day No-Cooking Diet*	Total Fitness for Women-U.S. Edition*
7-Day Diet for Women*	Total Fitness for Women - Metric
7-Day Diet for Men*	Total Fitness for Women - UK Edition
7-Day No-Cooking Diets*	Total Fitness for Men - U.S. Edition*
90-Day Gluten-Free Diet-1200 Cal*	Total Fitness for Men- Metric Edition*
90-Day Gluten-Free Diet-1500 Cal*	Total Fitness for Men - UK Edition
30-Day Gluten-Free Quick Diet*	Senior Fitness - U.S. Edition*
30-Day Gluten-Free No-Cooking Diet*	Senior Fitness - Metric Edition*
7-Day Diet for Women - Metric*	Senior Fitness - UK Edition*
7-Day Diet for Men - Metric	Computer Diet - U.S. Edition*
7-Day Gluten-Free Express Diet*	Computer Diet - Metric Edition*
7-Day Gluten-Free No-Cooking Diet*	Reliable Weight Loss - U.S. Edition
90-Day Vegetarian Diet-1200 Calorie*	Reliable Weight Loss - Metric Edition
90-Day Vegetarian Diet-1500 Calorie*	101 Weight Loss Tips*
30-Day Vegetarian Diet*	101 Healthy Eating Tips*
7-Day Vegetarian Diet*	101 Lifelong Fitness Tips*
Weight Loss for Women*	101 Weight Maintenance Tips
Weight Loss for Women - Metric	101 Weight Loss Recipes
Weight Loss for Women - UK	101 Gluten-Free Weight Loss Recipes
Weight Loss for Men*	101 Vegetarian Weight Loss Recipes*
Maximum Weight Loss - 1200 Cal	90-Day Mediterranean Diet - 1200 Cal
Maximum Weight Loss - 1500 Cal	90-Day Mediterranean Diet - 1500 Cal

* These titles are available as both ebooks and paperbacks.
NoPaperPress ebooks sold by Amazon, Apple, Google, Barnes & Noble and Kobo.
NoPaperPress paperbacks are only sold by Amazon.

Disclaimer

This book offers general exercise, information. It is not a medical manual and the author does not claim to be medically qualified. The material in this book is not intended to be a substitute for medical counseling. Everyone should have a medical checkup before beginning a physical fitness program (whether the program involves weight loss, nutritional changes, or exercise). Moreover, the physician conducting the medical exam should be made aware of and should approve the specific physical fitness routine planned. Further, the reader is cautioned that all fitness programs include some risk of injury or illness. Additionally, while the author and publisher have made every effort to ensure the accuracy of the information in this book, they make no representations or warranties regarding its accuracy or completeness. Further, neither the author nor publisher assume liability for any medical problems that might result from applying the methods in this book, or for any loss of profit, or any other commercial damages, including but not limited to special, incidental, consequential or other damages, and any such liability is hereby expressly disclaimed.

Earl Simmons is a personal trainer and free-lance health writer. He lives in Canada with his wife and two children.